# INSULIN USES & ABUSES

# INSULIN USES & ABUSES

Val Wilson

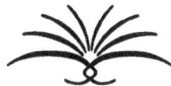

CAMBRIA
PRESS

Amherst, New York

Library of Congress Control Number: 2014958597

Wilson, Val.
Insulin Uses and Abuses .
p. cm.
Includes bibliographical references and index.
ISBN 978-1-934844-63-2 (alk. paper).

*For Neil*

# TABLE OF CONTENTS

# Introduction

Insulin is a hormone that everybody needs, but problems arise when there is too much or too little of it. It is responsible for many functions in the body, but the most well-known of these is to regulate blood glucose levels. In addition, insulin enables the synthesis of proteins; it changes the activity of many of the body's enzymes; it forces cells to absorb potassium, lowering the level in the bloodstream; it enables the artery walls to relax, encouraging blood flow; it causes the stomach to secrete hydrochloric acid in response to food; and it plays a role in the excretion of sodium in the urine. This hard-working hormone can also put someone in a coma and can even kill in the right circumstances.

Insulin was first discovered in 1921 and from its commercial availability in 1922 onwards, it has been responsible for miraculously changing the lives of people with Type 1 diabetes, lifting their former death sentence from the condition. However, unless insulin levels are closely monitored, too much insulin can lead to unconsciousness and too little can trigger the development of chronic and life-threatening complications such as heart and kidney disease. In 1927 insulin was first used as a method of committing suicide; in 1956 insulin became a murder weapon in the belief that, as a natural substance produced by the body, it could not be traced.

Numerous other instances of insulin being involved in single or even multiple unnatural deaths have occurred since, and determining the use of insulin in the crime has always been difficult, but it has been achieved.

## ABOUT THIS BOOK

Because insulin is such a powerful hormone, its potential for use and abuse is extensive. It has many vital roles, meaning major disruption when something goes wrong with the body's glucose regulation system. This can be altered following several night's of poor sleep and, if this continues, it is even possible that Type 2 diabetes may develop. This book begins by exploring the role of insulin in the body, and what happens when this is disrupted by disease, infection, hormonal variations, sleep disturbance, and certain medications. Historically, insulin has also been used as a "treatment" for schizophrenia and addiction in the belief that, by plunging non-diabetic individuals into severe unconsciousness with massive doses of insulin, this depletion of glucose for the brain would jolt it into working normally. Needless to say, this barbaric treatment was eventually discontinued, but it took forty years to admit that insulin coma therapy did not actually work.

Because insulin can act as a powerful anabolic agent to build muscle (creating larger molecules from smaller ones), this action has been seized upon, especially in recent years, by athletes. Insulin has been used, often in combination with other hormones and substances, to build muscle which cannot be easily broken down, meaning that some sportspersons have an edge over their competitors. There are many different types of insulin and the majority cannot be tested for, meaning that insulin has been a banned substance in sport since 1998, except for athletes with Type 1 diabetes who are prescribed the hormone for medical use. The abuse of insulin is unfortunately not confined to misguided medical treatments or sporting cheats. For some with Type 1 diabetes, restricting or omitting their insulin can be a way of losing weight very quickly. This practice, known as diabulimia, is not recognised as a medical condition, but is thought to be occurring in as many as one in three young females who need to treat their diabetes with regular insulin administration. This book provides unique insight into those who have experienced diabulimia, including how this began, how it ended, the consequences, and the help that can be offered to sufferers.

Insulin is thought to be an untraceable murder weapon, and as such, it has been the substance of choice for almost sixty years for a number of nurses (and one psychiatrist) who had easy access to this hormone. The cases that have been documented are many and this goes right up to present day, where a nurse was charged in March 2014 on three counts of murder using insulin. Because diabetes and hypoglycaemia also have great potential for fiction writers, insulin murder and unconsciousness are often portrayed for dramatic effect on television and in books and films. The ways in which the power of insulin is shown in fiction is also explored. However, getting the correct information across to the viewer or reader is sometimes sadly lacking.

# Insulin Uses & Abuses

# Chapter One

# The production and use of insulin by the body

Insulin is a polypeptide hormone (a chemical messenger) and a protein produced by the pancreas. The pancreas itself is both an endocrine and exocrine gland, meaning it is a ductless gland that secretes hormones into the bloodstream (its endocrine action); and a gland that secretes hormones into ducts that empty into epithelial tissue or directly into a body cavity (its exocrine action). The pancreas is a six-inch long organ extending across the abdomen and consists of a head, body and tail with a number of functions relating to the digestion of food. The exocrine part of the pancreas secretes pancreatic amylase which breaks downs starchy foods; trypsin to digest protein; and pancreatic lipase to break down triglycerides into fatty acids.

Dispersed among the exocrine portions constituting 98 percent of the mass of the pancreas are two to three million tiny clusters of hormone-producing cells known as the islets of Langerhans (Tortora and Grabowski, 1993). These were first discovered by Paul Langerhans, a medical student, who published his research dissertation in 1869 on the structure of the "pancreatic islands" (the islets of Langerhans) he had observed under the microscope, although he initially mistook these islets for lymph glands (Islam, 2000). Langerhans had also discovered that the pancreas contains nine types of cells, one of which secreted pancreatic juice (enzymes), another secreting "an unknown substance", the purpose of which was later identified and named as insulin by Banting and Best in 1921 (Banting and Best, 1922; Banting, 1929). At post mortem examination, people who have had diabetes are found to have a shrivelled pancreas due to altered insulin-producing cells, where the organ is comprised of fibrous tissue and often stones are present in the pancreatic ducts.

The islets of the pancreas do not just secrete insulin but are comprised of four types of hormone-secreting cells: the alpha cells secreting the hormone glucagon which raises blood glucose levels when it falls too low or when there is insufficient glucose available to maintain normal blood glucose levels; the beta cells which, as seen previously, secrete insulin to lower blood glucose levels; the delta cells which secrete growth hormone-inhibiting hormone, also known as somastostatin, which works to inhibit the secretion of insulin and glucagon when necessary; and the F-cells which secrete a polypeptide to regulate the release of the digestive enzymes amylase, trypsin and lipase (Tortora and Grabowski, 1993). The islet cells have a rich blood supply and are surrounded by clusters of exocrine cells known as acini.

Glucagon, released by the alpha cells of the pancreas, increases blood glucose levels as a protective measure for the brain and vital organs to provide them with fuel when there is too much insulin present in the bloodstream and hypoglycaemia results. Glucagon attaches to the liver cells to make them release stored glucose quickly into the bloodstream. Glucagon accelerates the conversion of stored glucose (glycogen) in the liver into a usable form of glucose, a process known as glycogenolysis, and also promotes the formation of glucose from lactic acid and certain amino acids in a process, known as gluconeogenesis, therefore enabling the release of glucose into the blood (Tortora and Grabowski, 1993). The release of both insulin when blood glucose levels are too high (hyperglycaemia) and glucagon when levels fall too low (hypoglycaemia) is regulated by the concentration of glucose in the blood in a negative feedback system. When blood glucose levels are detected as being low the alpha islet cells secrete more glucagon and once blood glucose levels are raised to normal levels (between 4.0–7.0mmol/L or 72 to 126 mg/dl American measurement) this action diminishes, although this process can continue until a state of excessive hyperglycaemia is reached.

This counter-regulation of blood glucose levels does not occur in the case of diabetes, as the pancreatic beta cells do not produce insulin, or only a small amount, due to auto-immune attack on the insulin-producing cells (Type 1 diabetes); or too much insulin is produced but cannot be used effectively if there is excess body fat impeding its function on cells (Type 2 diabetes). In Type 1 diabetes, when there is hypoglycaemia due to the injection of too much insulin, or unexpected exertion, the liver triggers the release of glucagon as a counter-regulatory measure to prevent damage to the brain from reduced glucose levels. However, as sometimes occurs in non-diabetic individuals, because the alpha cells continue to raise the blood glucose level, severe hyperglycaemia results (>15mmol/L or >270mg/dl). Other factors causing the release of glucagon by the alpha cells of the pancreas into the bloodstream in those with and without diabetes are the consumption of high-protein meals which raise the amino acid level of the blood, and increased activity of the autonomic nervous system during strenuous exercise (Tortora and Grabowski, 1993). Both insulin and glucagon can attach to any cell in the body, where they work, before being rapidly removed in the bloodstream.

Glycogen is a stored form of energy which is very useful in the short-term, but if there is a long-term lack of food, for example when an individual is dieting or when food is in short supply, fat stores in the tissues are utilised as a source of fuel (Sonksen and Sonksen, 2000). Fat can be substituted as an energy source instead of glucose in most, but not all tissues; muscle tissue readily moves from glucose to fat once glucose stores are depleted. However the brain and neural tissues can only use glucose for fuel (Cranston, 2005) but can substitute ketones (the waste products of protein metabolism) for the majority of their energy needs (Sonksen and Sonksen, 2000). Protein is also synthesised and broken down to be used as fuel when glycogen stores are low, a process called proteolysis. This process is inhibited by the presence of insulin in the bloodstream and when there is a lack of insulin, such as at the onset of Type 1 diabetes prior to treatment, ketoacidosis occurs. This is a serious condition where the level of ketone bodies in the blood rises to dangerous levels which adversely alter the tight parameters of acidity of the body.

Ketoacidosis is an acute and significant complication of Type 1 diabetes that occurs when the blood glucose level becomes consistently very high (>15mmol/L or >270mg/dl) causing the breakdown of fats as an alternative source of energy to glucose that cannot be easily used in the lack of insulin. This causes extreme and rapid weight loss, being the basis of high-protein diets, and is worryingly sometimes induced by those prescribed insulin for Type 1 diabetes in a condition called diabulimia to achieve weigh loss quickly by omitting insulin or by giving a deliberately small and incorrect dose (Wilson, 2012). Predominantly in people with Type 1 diabetes, (although people with Type 2 diabetes may also need to take insulin and may suffer from ketoacidosis), ketoacidosis is frequently seen due to forgetting to inject insulin or under-dosing, especially during illness when insulin needs can increase three-fold due to infection (Jarvis and Rubin, 2003).

Ketoacidosis is the major cause of mortality in people with Type 1 diabetes because the condition leads to circulatory collapse, low serum potassium levels and swelling of the brain, known as cerebral oedema (Katsilambros et al, 2011). A state of ketoacidosis can also occur in people with and without diabetes at times when the body's need for insulin is increased, such as during illness or physical stress. Other potential causes are pregnancy in females of childbearing age; the condition may also be associated with trauma, myocardial infarction (heart attack), congestive heart failure, cerebrovascular accident (stroke), gastrointestinal bleeding and undiagnosed diabetes (Russell, 2012).

## THE FORMATION AND DEGRADATION OF INSULIN

The human insulin molecule is a peptide hormone that is composed of 51 amino acids and is encoded in the INS gene (Bell et al, 1980). Pro-insulin is the molecule from which insulin is made by the beta cells of the pancreas. It can be detected and measured in the blood when the concentration of insulin is very high due to over-production by the pancreas, but not when insulin has been injected. The level of pro-insulin is tested when it is necessary to determine whether there has been malicious administration of insulin into a person suffering with severe hypoglycaemia (Marks and Richmond, 2007). Pro-insulin undergoes maturation into active insulin due to the action of cellular peptidases in a process of pro-hormone conversion. A second substance, C-peptide, is an essential but biologically inactive building block that is formed during insulin manufacture in the beta cells of the pancreas. C-peptide is made by the pancreas when it produces insulin and is stored in the insulin-producing cells until both are released into the bloodstream in response to a rise in blood glucose levels in non-diabetic individuals. Low blood glucose levels due to malnutrition or alcoholism are associated with a low level of C-peptide (Marks and Richmond, 2007).

Exogenous (injected) insulin is associated with a low or absent level of C-peptide. This is because this insulin is not produced by the pancreatic beta cells, so accompanying C-peptide would not be present in a person with Type 1 insulin-dependent diabetes as they do not produce any of their own insulin. Absence of C-peptide during a test to determine whether insulin has been maliciously administered can prove that any insulin present is pharmaceutical, rather than naturally secreted, and that it has therefore been injected. The insulin to C-peptide ratio tends to be 6:1 meaning 6x as much C-peptide as insulin is present in living people and a ratio of 20:1 after death (Marks and Richmond, 2007). If a very low blood glucose level is caused by the injection of insulin, the plasma insulin level will be high, but the plasma C-peptide level will be low as the insulin is not naturally secreted.

Insulin and C-peptide levels in the blood behave very differently from one another and it is possible for a person's blood to contain one without the other (Marks and Richmond, 2007). The level of C-peptides present in the urine of a person with Type 1 diabetes can indicate the level of insulin-producing beta cell function to determine if there is any function remaining, leading to a better prognosis for the individual (Marks and Richmond, 2007). Urine C-peptide level however bears no relation to blood C-peptide level. Once the insulin molecule has been formed in the beta cells, the resulting mature insulin then waits for metabolic signals from substances in the bloodstream such as leucine, arginine, glucose and mannose. The mature insulin molecule also receives autonomic nerve signals from the vagus nerve to stimulate the insulin to function as it reaches the target area of the cell where it begins the action of reducing glucose.

Following completion of its task, the insulin molecule may return to the extracellular environment outside the cell wall or the cell using the insulin molecule may render it inactive, a process known as degradation which occurs approximately one hour after the insulin molecule enters the blood circulation (Duckworth et al, 1999). Insulin is also cleared from the bloodstream by the liver when the insulin contained in the blood passes through the hepatic blood vessels, and in a secondary process by the kidneys via the systemic circulation of the blood. A high plasma insulin level therefore does not equate to a low blood glucose level (Marks and Richmond, 2007) as it may be inactive insulin in the process of being cleared from the body. The proteins which make up the insulin molecule have now been located within the brain and research has shown that a deficiency in these proteins is associated with the onset of Altzheimer's disease (de la Monte et al, 2005; Steen et al, 2005).

## THE MANY FUNCTIONS OF INSULIN

As previously mentioned, insulin has the opposite action of glucagon in lowering blood glucose levels. Insulin has a number of actions in the body (Tortora and Grabowski, 1993):

- Insulin causes the cells of the liver, skeletal muscle and fat cells to absorb glucose from the blood for fuel. Glucose is stored in the liver as glycogen; in muscle, and in the fat cells (adipocytes) it is stored as triglycerides.
- Insulin decreases glucose uptake in non-skeletal muscle. This is the case because the trigger for glucose uptake by muscle tissue is hyperglycaemia, as well as the concentration between intracellular and extracellular glucose levels (Sonksen and Sonksen, 2000).
- With the exception of those with either Type 1 or Type 2 diabetes, the secretion of insulin to maintain normal levels of blood glucose prevents glucose building up in the bloodstream to what becomes a toxic level (hyperglycaemia).
- Insulin promotes the entry of amino acids into the body cells and enables the synthesis of proteins. Acting as a metabolic control, insulin regulates body systems such as anabolic effects (the production of molecules) and amino acid uptake. Amino acid uptake, controlled by insulin, increases DNA replication.
- Insulin enables the conversion of glucose and other nutrients into fatty acids in the process of lipogenesis. Therefore, insulin enables fat stores to be laid down.
- The hormone insulin promotes the conversion of excess glucose to glycogen in the process of glycogenesis.
- The hormone insulin decreases the process of glycogenolysis, where the liver stores excess glucose as glycogen.
- Insulin also slows the process of glyconeogenesis, the conversion of stored glycogen back into glucose where it is released into the bloodstream.
- Insulin changes the activity of many of the body's enzymes.

- By increasing potassium uptake, insulin forces body cells to absorb serum potassium thereby lowering potassium levels in the bloodstream.

- Insulin forces the walls of arteries to be relaxed in order to increase blood flow. This is especially the case for smaller arteries and with less insulin, these arteries are forced to contract, reducing blood flow.

- The presence of insulin causes the parietal cells in the stomach to secrete hydrochloric acid to aid the digestion of food.

- Insulin causes the kidneys to excrete less sodium in the urine (Gupta et al, 1992). This means that a higher level is retained in the body with the potential of raising blood pressure levels.

- The presence of insulin in the brain, once it has entered via the bloodstream, has been shown to enhance memory, learning and cognition, especially verbal cognition in particular (Benedict et al, 2004). However, Marks and Richmond (2007) have stated that the brain does not contain or produce any insulin. It would appear that, as the brain is supplied with blood, any insulin in the bloodstream would thus also be present in the brain.

- Research using nasal insulin to enhance the level of insulin present in the brain has shown a beneficial increase for healthy, non-diabetic individuals in thermoregulation (control of body temperature) and glucoregulation (how the body responds to glucose intake from food) suggesting that the amount of insulin present in the central nervous system helps regulate homeostasis (the regulation of body energy) in humans (Benedict et al, 2010).

The release of insulin (with the exception of those individuals with Type 1 diabetes) or glucagon into the bloodstream is regulated by the blood glucose level. Increased amounts of certain amino acids and hormones, such as human growth hormone (which has an impact on glucose regulation) in the bloodstream, also stimulate the secretion of insulin. This impact on glucose regulation is one of the reasons why Type 1 diabetes can be very difficult to manage in adolescence (Tasker et al, 2007), and due to hormonal changes, puberty can lead to frequent hyperglycaemia (Amiel et al, 1986; Hanas, 2006). Insulin is also released following stimulation of the parasympathetic division of the autonomic nervous system in response to eating (Tortora and Grabowski, 1993).

When there is a high level of insulin in the bloodstream, the ovaries are stimulated to release testosterone in response (Marks and Richmond, 2007), which is the male sex hormone, stimulating the production of sperm and developing and maintaining the appearance of male characteristics. Therefore frequent severe episodes of hypoglycaemia in females with Type 1 diabetes can be associated with the development of characteristics such as excess facial hair as a consequence of continually high levels of insulin in the bloodstream. A rapid fall in blood glucose levels due to the action of insulin is also associated with a sharp increase in the level of adrenaline present in the bloodstream, a technique employed by drug addicts to get a high (Marks and Richmond, 2007), although this is dangerous to drug users and people with Type 1 diabetes as adrenaline increases the heart rate. A relationship between insulin and other hormone levels is also seen when there is an elevated level of thyroid hormone in the blood; this raises blood glucose levels by reducing the amount of insulin secreted by the beta cells (Jarvis and Rubin, 2003).

## DISORDERS OF INSULIN PRODUCTION

For several years prior to the diagnosis of Type 1 diabetes, the individual's immune system releases proteins into the blood which are islet cell antibodies. This shows that Type 1 diabetes is an autoimmune disease where the body effectively attacks the pancreatic beta cells, impairing their insulin production function. In addition, treatments to reduce this autoimmunity status have been shown to delay the onset of Type 1 diabetes (Jarvis and Rubin, 2003), and those who develop the condition also tend to also have other autoimmune diseases such as asthma or hypothyroidism (an under active thyroid gland). When there is insufficient insulin being produced due to autoimmune attack, Type 1 diabetes results, leading to a state of hyperglycaemia (high blood glucose levels), where the body cells cannot easily use the rising amount of glucose as fuel without insulin as a catalyst.

The characteristics of Type 1 diabetes being caused by the body's own immune system attacking the insulin-producing beta cells of the pancreas is now thought to be triggered by a virus. Exposure to this virus in the environment which directly attacks the pancreas and cannot be fought off due to a weakened immune system creates the diabetic state (Jarvis and Rubin, 2003). This attack cannot be reversed and Type 1 diabetes is a permanent chronic condition requiring insulin to be replaced by several daily injections or with the use of insulin pump therapy which provides continuous insulin delivery under the skin and additional programmed dosages for food or when more insulin is required (Wilson, 2003). However, as previously mentioned, there are two types of diabetes, both resulting in hyperglycaemia when untreated but having different causes.

In addition to Type 1 diabetes, if the body is unable to use glucose appropriately in the presence of excess body fat, large amounts of insulin are produced in an attempt to reduce blood glucose levels that cannot be used as the action of insulin is impaired by fat. This results in high blood glucose levels and eventually, Type 2 diabetes. The symptoms of both Type 1 and Type 2 are similar because they are both due to high levels of glucose in the body: excessive urination and excessive thirst, which is the body's attempt to flush out the glucose it cannot use as fuel as a waste product. Untreated Type 1 diabetes leads to rapid weight loss because the body then utilises fat and protein as a source of fuel in the absence of insulin (a state of ketoacidosis). It has now been recognised that Type 2 diabetes can go undiagnosed for up to 12 years because the onset of symptoms are not as dramatic and rapid as in Type 1 diabetes (World Health Organisation, 2011; Diabetes UK, 2008).

Symptoms such as tiredness, frequent urination, blurred vision, slow healing of wounds, numbness in the feet and legs, and obesity may be tolerated by the individual for many years before consulting a doctor, or where blood glucose is checked routinely and found to be high. However, complications of diabetes due to high and continual blood glucose levels, such as eye, heart or kidney disease may have already begun before diagnosis of the primary condition. There are now also cases of children, traditionally only developing Type 1 diabetes, who are now developing Type 2 due to physical inactivity and obesity; the same cause as in adults (Wilson, 2013).

Gestational diabetes during pregnancy may also occur because of the hormones produced by the placenta and growing foetus (from week 20 of the pregnancy) so that it can develop correctly. This surge in hormones from the baby entering the mother's body results in hyperglycaemia in the mother due to reduced insulin sensitivity. This leads to symptoms similar to those of Type 2 diabetes (World Health Organisation, 2011). If uncontrolled, high blood glucose levels also cross the placenta from mother to baby, resulting in a larger amniotic sac surrounding the foetus (filled with the baby's urine and fluid waste products) and also heavier babies. This type of diabetes occurs in around 2 percent of all pregnancies and actual Type 2 diabetes develops approximately 15 years later in more than half of women who have had gestational diabetes. The reason is thought to be due to genetic susceptibility to diabetes in these women and the level of glucagon (the anti-insulin hormone) present during pregnancy (Jarvis and Rubin, 2003).

## HYPERGLYCAEMIA

As mentioned earlier, when there is a lack of, or insufficient insulin present in the body, hyperglycaemia or high blood glucose levels result. As previously seen, this condition can be dangerous and is classed as a medical emergency in association with an increase in the body's acidity level when there is diabetic ketoacidosis (Russell, 2012; Katsilambros et al, 2011). If blood glucose levels are continually raised over time due to untreated or poorly managed Type 1 or Type 2 diabetes, chronic diabetic complications eventually develop due to the body's reaction to large amounts of glucose in the cells which is toxic and cannot be effectively dealt with.

A further potential cause of chronic diabetic complications relates to the way glucose is metabolised by the body. As energy is produced, carbon dioxide and water are released but, in the presence of large amounts of glucose which impairs the function of cells, it is metabolised into sorbitol (Barnett and Grice, 2011). This substance accumulates in the body's tissues and causes damage as the osmotic pressure (fluid balance) inside and outside the cells is equalised and because the sorbitol cannot pass through the cell membrane and becomes trapped. This results in damage and destruction to body cells (but sorbitol used as an artificial sweetener does not have this effect in the body). These complex metabolic processes and the continual presence of excessive glucose appear to be a causative factor in the development of chronic complications. It is also understood that genetic factors may lead to complications for individuals with diabetes, even in those people who maintain their blood glucose levels within normal limits (Barnett and Grice, 2011).

Diabetes is a multi-system disease which affects all areas of the body because if blood glucose levels are high, all cells and tissues are damaged by the toxicity of excess glucose. Chronic secondary complications of diabetes are many and may take up to 10 years to develop after a long period of poor blood glucose control (Shaw and Cummings, 2005), even developing over time in those who have relatively stable diabetes control. This may be because of the altered metabolic state in diabetes meaning that complications are inevitable over time because normal body processes are altered by the disease. Poorly-controlled diabetes is therefore associated with sight impairment, kidney disease, nerve damage, micro-vascular (small blood vessels) and macro-vascular disease affecting the large blood vessels and heart.

This was proven beyond any doubt for those with Type 1 diabetes in the Diabetes Control and Complications Trial (DCCT), 1993; and for Type 2 diabetes in the UK Prospective Diabetes Study (UKPDS), 1998.

Both studies showed that high blood glucose levels due to undiagnosed or poorly managed diabetes (including those people with Type 1 whose diabetes is very difficult to control with insulin), leads to the development of and the worsening of existing chronic complications. However, some individuals have a greater tolerance for raised glucose levels in the blood and appear to escape the development of complications, despite seemingly difficult to manage or poor glycaemic (blood glucose) control. Despite these groundbreaking studies showing this definitive link between poor glycaemic control and the development of chronic complications, the exact percentage of glucose present in the blood which will actually trigger complications to develop in the body is not defined. These studies suggest that maintaining a blood glucose percentage (HbA1c) level of 6.5 percent for those without complications and 6.0 percent for those already with complications will slow the development or progression of the chronic health problems associated with diabetes.

It is known that certain medications and nutritional supplements adversely affect blood glucose levels. Secretion of insulin is suppressed by nicotinic acid or niacin (vitamin B3) taken in a vitamin supplement or prescribed to treat high levels of cholesterol, with the effect of raising blood glucose levels. Thiazide diuretics often increase the level of glucose in the blood by causing loss of potassium in the urine (Jarvis and Rubin, 2003). This is also the case for many medications prescribed to treat high blood pressure: beta blockers such as Atenolol and Bisopropol; and Minoxidil; calcium channel blockers such as Nifedipine and Amlodipine (Jarvis and Rubin, 2003). Corticosteroids, even in the form of a topical steroid cream, can raise blood glucose levels. This is also true of Cyclosporine, Prednisone, Immuran and Tacrolimus tablets, taken to prevent organ rejection after transplant, as they poison the insulin-producing beta cells (Robertson et al, 1988). Phenothiazines (anti-psychotic drugs) such as Chlorpromazine, Promazine, Fluphenazine, Tripfluoperzaine, and Thioridazine (now not used in the UK), are also known to block the secretion of insulin, causing hyperglycaemia.

Maintaining normal glycaemic control (normoglycaemia) with the correct amount of insulin administered by injection or insulin pump (exogenous insulin rather than that produced by the beta cells), or glucose-reducing medications is the key to avoiding the development of chronic diabetic complications. This may not always be possible, for example, when insulin requirements are raised due to infection. Normoglycaemia achieved when possible means delaying or avoiding hyperglycaemia which can lead to:

- Blindness because the sensitive blood vessels in the eyes can burst or leak; cataracts form where the lenses in the eyes becomes cloudy; and retinopathy develops due to damage at the back of the eye.

- Kidney failure due to the kidneys filtering urine containing large glucose molecules which harden and disrupt the function of the nephrons.

- Heart disease and stroke because the blood becomes thickened due to its glucose content and due to fatty deposits narrowing the arteries.

- Amputation due to reduced blood supply to the limbs and because of slow wound healing.

In 2011 the World Health Organisation estimated that 364 million people worldwide had diabetes (90 percent of cases being Type 2) and stated that in 2004, an estimated 3.4 million people died from the chronic complications of the disease (WHO, 2011). Diabetes raises the risk of heart disease and stroke because of hyperglycaemia and 50 percent of people with diabetes die from cardiovascular causes or stroke. Reduced blood flow and nerve damage (present in 50 percent of people with diabetes) significantly increases the risk of lower limb amputation and ulceration of the feet and lower legs for people with diabetes. After a 15-year duration of diabetes approximately two percent of people with diabetes lose their sight and 10 percent develop a substantial visual impairment. In addition, 10–20 percent of people with diabetes die from kidney failure. Because diabetes has the potential to damage every part of the body because high levels of blood glucose are transported to every living tissue, a person with poorly-managed diabetes with frequent hyperglycaemia is twice as likely to die than a person without the condition (WHO, 2011). Chronic complications are, in conjunction with the prevalence of the primary disease, especially the ever-escalating number of people developing Type 2 diabetes in the world, the reason why diabetes is such a major health issue annually costing billions to treat.

## TYPES OF HYPOGLYCAEMIA

The symptoms of hypoglycaemia: confusion, irritability, weakness/shakiness, hunger, headache and tiredness, are similar to the body's reaction to stress and anxiety and lead to catecholamine release by the adrenal glands (Tortora and Grabowski, 1993). Catecholamines increase blood glucose levels by triggering the release of glucagon by the liver to rapidly increase blood glucose levels providing necessary fuel for the "fight or flight" response. There are several different ways in which low blood glucose levels manifest due to an excess of insulin (Wilson, 2011). A person suffering from hypoglycaemia who is cold will lose their shivering reflex and a combination of alcohol and shivering lead to hypothermia. Although almost all cases of severe hypoglycaemia are reversible with the speedy administration of glucagon by injection into a vein (or muscle), or glucose by mouth if the individual is not unconscious, in rare cases of irreversible hypoglycaemia, the individual cannot respond to pain (Marks and Richmond, 2007). A rapid fall in blood glucose levels is accompanied by a fall in blood potassium level that triggers the release of glucagon, cortisol and adrenaline (epinephrine) as the body attempts to quickly raise glucose levels to protect the functions of the brain and the heart.

Increased levels of blood insulin may also trigger the release of anti-diuretic hormone (ADH) to help adrenaline and glucose to raise blood glucose levels, in addition to inhibiting the production of urine (Marks and Richmond, 2007). A sudden surge of epinephrine (adrenaline) into the bloodstream causes constriction of the blood vessels, an increase in blood pressure, heart rate and the force of cardiac contractions, putting a lethal strain on the heart. For this reason, prolonged severe hypoglycaemia can lead to cardiac arrhythmia and multiple organ failure (Marks and Richmond, 2007). The symptoms of severe hypoglycaemia are predominantly neuropsychiatric and a state of suspended animation may occur due to massive cerebral shock, causing cognitive impairment, loss of communication, paralysis of all four limbs, and double incontinence. However, the patient's eyes remain open and breathing continues despite drastically low blood glucose levels, with the hypothalamic and brainstem reflexes still active (Kaufman, 2007). Hypoglycaemia can occur naturally in individuals suffering from liver and kidney disease, thought to be associated with the use of bicarbonate-based substitution fluid during continuous venous haemofiltration (dialysis), poor nutrition due to lack of appetite, and sepsis (Vriesendorp et al, 2006).

Reactive hypoglycaemia results when there is a physiological over-compensation of insulin (where the body produces too much) in non-diabetic individuals. Hypoglycaemia can result if there is a large amount of glucose present in food or drink, and this can occur up to four hours after eating causing the blood glucose level to fall to <3.9mmol/L (<70mg/dl). This may be due to a number of reasons. Islet hyperplasia is a condition where the alpha islet cells producing glucagon and the beta islet cells producing insulin are uniformly enlarged because of an increase in the number of alpha cells rather than beta cells, thought to be due to changes in glycogen secretion. This type of hypoglycaemia is common in people with an insulin-secreting tumour (insulinoma) of the pancreas and insulin hyperplasia is rarely the cause of undetected hypoglycaemia (Patti et al, 2005).

Autoimmune syndrome results in a high concentration of insulin in the blood despite low blood glucose levels. The insulin produced is mostly inactive as it is strongly bound to antibodies in blood plasma, although this can reverse so the insulin becomes active. Where the action of insulin is impaired by antibodies, the blood glucose level rapidly rises following a meal which causes more insulin to be secreted. The antibodies do not bind well to C-peptide, released when insulin is produced, causing insulin to disappear from the bloodstream at the normal rate. This means that there is an elevated level of plasma insulin in people with a low C-peptide level and an accompanying positive level of anti-insulin antibodies (Cavaco et al, 2001).

Glycogen storage disease may also lead to reactive hypoglycaemia in adults. In this condition, the enzyme which breaks down stored glycogen into glucose sub-units (phosphorylase) is faulty causing slow release of glucose by the liver and resulting hypoglycaemia. This can be tested by injecting glucagon, which normally stimulates the formation of phosphorylase sub-units and, if the release of glucose into the bloodstream is slow, glycogen storage disease is confirmed. The condition is managed by advising patients to eat slow-release carbodhydrates such as potatoes and pasta so that blood glucose levels do not rise rapidly (Miller et al, 2009). Gastric surgery can lead to reactive hypoglycaemia, originally thought to be the result of increased insulin production in response to excess body fat; the action of insulin being impaired by fat, this being the origin of Type 2 diabetes. However, more recent research has shown that this is not the case (Service et al, 2005) demonstrating that reactive hypoglycaemia following gastric band surgery is due to an acquired phenomenon or gastric dumping prompting increased insulin production after meals.

Fasting hypoglycaemia occurs in those without diabetes early in the morning after an overnight fast and is common when dieting, or following vigorous exercise, causing the blood glucose level to fall as low as 3mmol/L (54mg/dl). This condition may also be caused by a benign insulin-producing tumour, and rarely by breast or adrenal cancer, which triggers the release of insulin-like growth factor II. In addition, fasting hypoglycaemia may be due to the consumption of a moderately large amount of alcohol (especially on an empty stomach), occurring two to five hours later (Chow and Chow, 2007); although a reduction in blood glucose can occur after drinking as little as 150ml of whisky (Marks and

Richmond, 2007). Different types of alcohol, for example, beer rather than whisky, may reduce the blood glucose level at different rates determined by the carbohydrate content of the drink, although alcohol (altering metabolic rate) does not reduce blood glucose levels in the same way as insulin (allowing glucose to be used as fuel by the cells). Studies have demonstrated that chronic alcoholism can lead to transient carbohydrate intolerance which has been recognised as a factor in the early development of Type 2 diabetes as it inhibits glyconeogenesis, the conversion of stored glycogen back into glucose, releasing it into the bloodstream (Huang and Sjőholm, 2008). Alcohol-induced hypoglycaemia damages the brain to a greater extent than insulin-induced hypoglycaemia and is more likely to lead to death (Marks and Richmond, 2007).

Medications can reduce blood glucose levels in the same way as with fasting hypoglycaemia, such as some forms of antibiotics, diuretics (some causing hyperglycaemia), corticosteroids (some with potential to also raise blood glucose levels), heroin, and barbiturates (George et al, 2005). Hypoglycaemia may also be caused by salicylates (aspirin and drugs derived from aspirin), especially when taken in large doses as these medications can increase the effects of blood glucose-lowering drugs taken to control Type 2 diabetes. In the 1970s it was suggested that aspirin could be useful in helping to lower blood glucose levels, especially for those with Type 2 diabetes, as it has the action of inhibiting the absorption of glucose in the small intestine (Arvanitikis et al, 1977). In addition, it is now known that combinations of over-the-counter remedies, such as aspirin and fish oils, can be dangerous if taken together because Omega-3 fatty acids found in fish oils also have the same effect as aspirin in lowering blood glucose levels (Harvard Health Publications, 2011). Therefore, if taken together with glucose-reducing drugs or insulin and not monitored with regular blood glucose tests, fish oils and aspirin can reduce blood glucose levels enough to cause frequent hypoglycaemia.

Alpha-blockers (used to treat high blood pressure), such as Doxazosin, also have the action of lowering blood glucose levels, as do fibric acid derivatives (used to treat disorders of fat), such as Clofibrate or Bezafibrate (Jarvis and Rubin, 2003). Consistently very low and unexplained blood glucose levels may also be caused by an underlying abnormality such as an insulinoma, a benign insulin-secreting tumour (Marks and Richmond, 2007). Severe infection, such as pneumonia, may also lead to hypoglycaemia in the non-diabetic individual due to inadequate nutrition and increased uptake of glucose by the body in response to fighting the infection; infectious diseases do not stimulate insulin secretion, with the exception of malaria. An increased uptake of glucose by the body is also the case for individuals with liver disease who develop septicaemia leading to hypoglycaemia, also accompanied by a rapid fall in plasma albumin levels (Marks and Richmond, 2007). People with liver, kidney, or glandular disease may suffer from hypoglycaemia because the metabolism of glucose by the body is altered in these conditions. A severe and prolonged depletion of oxygen can also result in hypoglycaemia because this alters the way body cells metabolise glucose for fuel (Marks and Richmond, 2007).

Hypoglycaemia is a common occurrence in babies and children. Severe hypoglycaemia increases the size of the child's liver because of the accumulated storage of glucagon, for example, from a glucose intravenous infusion or due to natural synthesis of glucose in the blood (Wilson, 2011). An enlarged liver is also a sign of insulin overdose in infants (Marks and Richmond, 2007). Galactosaemia is a rare condition seen in children where the ability to process galactose (natural sugars found in milk) is impaired. The symptoms of this condition, seen in very young babies who have been fed milk for a few weeks, include vomiting, weight loss, and the development of cataracts (cloudiness in the lenses of the eyes). The child's liver may not release glycogen into the bloodstream, resulting in hypoglycaemia. Treatment is by introducing a milk-free diet and use of non milk-based formula (Harrison and Gibson, 2009).

Glycogen storage disease, also known as glycogen synthesis deficiency (GSD-0), is common in children as well as adults. The condition leads to fasting hypoglycaemia, ketoacidosis and low to normal levels of blood lactate and alanine. GSD-0 is characterised by moderately low stores of glycogen in the liver rather than an excess of glycogen being stored, and hypoglycaemia within a few hours of eating (Miller et al, 2009). This occurs because of the small amount of glycogen stored and the lack of available glycogen to be released and converted into glucose to raise blood glucose levels. Growth hormone deficiency disease also causes hypoglycaemia because growth hormone restricts the action of insulin on muscle and fat cells leading to increased sensitivity to insulin, forcing the pancreas to produce more insulin. Hormone treatment enables this condition to be reversed in affected children (Aimaretti et al, 1998).

Hereditary fructose disorder causes hypoglycaemia in children because the body cannot metabolise natural fruit sugar. Hypoglycaemia is accompanied by vomiting and seizures, leading to unconsciousness. The condition is treated by giving glucose to raise blood glucose levels and by adopting a fruit-free diet (Perheetupa et al, 2009). Hypoglycaemia is also caused by the condition, nesidioblastosis, a rare disorder characterised by the secretion of large amounts of insulin and C-peptide in children, but also there are high blood glucose levels (Service et al, 2005). The condition is treated with Diazoxide drugs and surgical removal of the pancreas.

## INSULINOMA

These are rare and known as neuroendocrine tumours as they are derived from the insulin-producing beta cells of the pancreas in the endocrine portion. However this type of tumour can, in extremely rare cases, develop outside of the pancreas, for example, as a carcinoma attached to the small intestine (Marks and Richmond, 2007). An insulinoma tumour is classed as functional because it produces insulin, the unpredictable release of insulin causing blood glucose levels to fall so that they are continually low at around 2.5mmol/L (45 mg/dl). The over-production of insulin (hyperinsulinism) due to this condition was first recognised in

1924 by Searle Harris (Harris, 1924), and the first surgical removal of an insulinoma tumour from the pancreas was later performed in 1929.

There is a higher predominance for onset of an insulin-secreting tumour in middle-aged woman than in men. Most insulinomas are benign and are contained within the pancreas itself, but in 10 percent of cases they are malignant and the tumour may spread (as a secondary tumour) to the liver by the time of diagnosis. As seen previously, a primary insulinoma may, very rarely, develop outside the pancreas as a carcinoma, containing insulin-secreting cells, arising from a part of the digestive tract (Marks and Richmond, 2007).

An insulin-secreting tumour is diagnosed following a 24–72 hour fast and periodic measurement of blood glucose, insulin and pro-insulin levels to determine episodes of hypoglycaemia. The production of insulin by an insulinoma may also be diagnosed using Tolbutamide used to stimulate the pancreas to produce insulin during a glucose tolerance test which, in a healthy person, temporarily reduces the concentration of glucose in the blood for two hours (Marks and Richmond, 2007). If an insulinoma is present however, the blood glucose level will continue to fall due to insulin produced by the tumour. The presence of a high level of plasma insulin and C-peptide also indicate an insulin-secreting tumour and this is not the case if plasma C-peptide levels are low or undetectable; very rarely is an insulinoma the cause of undetectable hypoglycaemia (Marks and Richmond, 2007). The characteristics of episodic hypoglycaemia, raised levels of insulin, pro-insulin and C-peptide, which are associated with the development of an insulinoma, are confirmed by ultrasound or M.R.I. (Magnetic Resonance Imaging) scans. Very rarely is an insulinoma detected by the use of an abdominal C.T. (Computed Tomography) scan (Marks and Richmond, 2007).

In addition to ultrasound and M.R.I. scans, angiographic techniques may be used to test for raised insulin levels in the body (known as a calcium infusion test). Using an angiography scan, a blood sample is directly taken from the hepatic vein (transporting blood from the liver to the heart) via a small cannula (tube) inserted into the femoral artery in the groin and guided by radiological techniques to the hepatic vein. The secretion of insulin by the pancreas can be stimulated by injecting calcium gluconate into the three arteries supplying the pancreas with blood (Doppman et al, 1995); this test being designed to localise the existence and position of an insulin-secreting tumour. If there is then a large secretion of insulin by the pancreas following this test, the beta cells are regarded as abnormal (Marks and Richmond, 2007), indicating the presence of an insulin-secreting tumour as the injected calcium blocks the release of insulin.

If, despite the injection of calcium into the arteries supplying the pancreas with blood, there is a rise in the concentration of insulin in the hepatic vein, an insulin-secreting tumour may be suspected in the tail of the pancreas (Marks and Richmond, 2007). However, it is usual that with this condition, a rise in plasma insulin occurs only after the artery supplying the tail of the pancreas has been injected, and not when either of the two other arteries supplying the rest of the pancreas is injected with calcium (Marks and Richmond, 2007).

Once an insulinoma is confirmed as being the underlying cause of hypoglycaemia it is determined whether the tumour can be surgically removed. Prior to surgery, or in the event that the tumour cannot be removed, frequent and unpredictable hypoglycaemia due to an insulin-producing tumour may be managed with the drug, Octreotide, which specifically blocks the secretion of insulin by the pancreas (Marks and Richmond, 2007). Diazoxide or somastostatin and calcium channel-blockers such as Nifedipine and Amlodipine are additional medications that are also used to block or reduce the secretion of insulin (raising blood glucose levels) in the case of an inoperable insulinoma (Sweetman, 2009). Patients experiencing periodic hypoglycaemia are also advised to eat little and often to reduce the action of insulin on blood glucose levels.

Permanent reversal of symptoms in operable cases is only achievable by surgical removal of the tumour where it may be necessary to also remove part of the pancreas as well. This is known as the Whipple procedure, named after Allen Whipple who successfully removed an insulin-secreting tumour in 1940 and described the symptoms and treatment of hypoglycaemia in 1938 (Johna and Schein, 2003). Because an insulinoma most commonly originates in the insulin-producing beta cells of the pancreas, removal of the majority or all of beta cells means that around two percent of patients go on to develop Type 1 diabetes and require daily insulin injections or continuous subcutaneous administration of insulin with insulin pump therapy as their own beta cells are no longer present. The procedure of removing the affected cells cures the vast majority of benign insulinoma tumours although multiple benign tumours may be present in the beta cells, causing continuing episodes of hypoglycaemia.

## INSULIN AND SLEEP

A century ago individuals got an average of nine hours' sleep per night; they now achieve an average of less than seven hours per night because of increasingly busy lifestyles, suggesting people around the world are now sleep-deprived (Sharma and Kavuru, 2010). Sleep involves a number of different and distinct stages during which the metabolic rate is temporarily altered. Following a phase of rapid eye movement (R.E.M.) sleep, a second phase of non-rapid eye movement (N.R.E.M.) sleep occurs. R.E.M. and N.R.E.M. sleep occurs in 90 minute cycles throughout the night (Siegel, 2003).This second phase is made up of four distinctive parts, the third and fourth of these being termed slow-wave sleep. Research has shown that during slow-wave sleep, the temperature of the brain is reduced and it is much less active than during other phases of sleep, allowing the metabolism to slow down by a rate of 15 percent (Goldberg et al, 1988; Brebbia and Autzhuler, 1965) in order that re-adjustment and repair of any damage occurring during waking hours can take place (Sharma and Kavuru, 2010).

The metabolic process (the way the body uses energy to maintain its functions) involves two stages: anabolism, when molecules are produced;

and catabolism, when molecules are broken down. These two biochemical processes maintain the energy requirements necessary for the normal working function of the body, for example, brain function, heart and respiratory function. It therefore follows that a lack of sleep can significantly interfere with metabolism, disrupting processes such as the storage of carbohydrates for fuel and the production of hormones, also adversely affecting cardiovascular function (Trennel, 2007).

In terms of the use of glucose by body cells, when the body has not had adequate sleep (eight hours according to Trennel, 2007), the level of thyroid-stimulating hormone released in response to metabolic rate is lowered. Thyroid stimulating hormone is responsible for stimulating the synthesis and secretion of thyroxin and triiodothyronine by the thyroid gland and for controlling basal and cellular metabolism, growth and development. The blood level of the hormone, cortisol, having an impact on glucose regulation, is also increased when there is a lack of sleep (Van Cauter et al, 1992). Cortisol is produced when the body is under stress, its action being to suppress the immune system and slow digestion at times when we react with our fight or flight response. Surges of cortisol and adrenaline (epinephrine), released when the body is stressed, kill off neurons in the hippocampus region of the brain, creating permanent memory loss (Wax, 2013).

For this reason, a reduction in sleep can also interfere with glucose metabolism causing a rise in blood glucose levels and (in non-diabetic individuals) the response by the beta cells of the pancreas to then release insulin to bring glucose levels back down to within the normal range. This over-stimulation of pancreatic beta cells to produce insulin in a yo-yo process of blood glucose levels rising and falling during sleep deprivation-induced metabolic disturbance can lead to Type 2 diabetes. A reduction in slow-wave sleep over as little as three nights has been shown to reduce insulin sensitivity in healthy subjects by 25 percent so that more insulin was necessary to reduce the same amount of blood glucose to a normal level (Sharma and Kavruru, 2010), a condition seen in those with impaired glucose tolerance eventually developing into Type 2 diabetes. Less than eight hours' sleep therefore adversely affects glucose tolerance and endocrine function.

The body has a remarkable capacity to bounce back following sleep loss, which is often unavoidable when, for example, a baby cries in the night, waking its parents, requiring attention. Studies have shown that this ability to do without as much sleep in the short term involves a rebound in metabolic function following slow-wave sleep loss and a spike in growth hormone in response to a reduction in levels following sleep loss (Sharma and Kavuru, 2010). However, when sleep loss is recurrent, the body eventually loses this ability to bounce back and there is no compensation for lack of short-wave sleep or disruption to the level of growth hormone in the blood (Spiegel et al, 2005; Spiegel et al, 2000).

This hormonal imbalance following sleep deprivation has also been shown with regard to glucose tolerance and insulin sensitivity (the cell's ability to use insulin correctly to reduce blood glucose levels), although this was only for one night and was corrected by the body following several nights of poor sleep (Van Cauter et al, 1997). Continual release of epinephrine and cortisol by the body when it is under stress due to lack of sleep eventually inhibits the action of the immune system. The hormone, serotonin, making us feel happy, is suppressed by the presence of epinephrine and cortisol and, over time, this can lead to serious illnesses such as depression, heart disease, hardening of the arteries, Type 2 diabetes and certain cancers (Wax, 2013).

As mentioned earlier, Type 2 diabetes comprises 90 percent of all cases of diabetes worldwide and the development of the condition has now reached epidemic proportions due to the trigger factor of the adoption by more societies of a Westernised diet (fast food, high in calories and fat) and an increasingly sedentary lifestyle. In London, United Kingdom alone, 1 in 20 people have now developed Type 2 diabetes (as at March 2013), with a further 250,000 individuals with insulin resistance (insulin insensitivity so the pancreas produces more to reduce blood glucose levels) whose diabetes is yet to develop. This figure has increased by 132,000 in London since March 2012, with the Department of Health currently spending 10 billion per year to treat and manage the condition and its chronic complications; it is estimated that this cost will rise to 17 billion pounds by 2025. Whilst not everyone who is over their ideal body weight will develop Type 2 diabetes, factors such as genetic inheritance and lifestyle will determine whether this is more likely in some than in others.

The inheritance of the genes for developing Type 2 diabetes are much stronger than those for developing Type 1 (Jarvis and Rubin, 2003). For a person with an identical twin who already has Type 2 diabetes, they have a 90 percent chance of also developing the condition at some point in their life; if one of the individual's parents has Type 2 diabetes, that person has a 40 percent chance of developing Type 2 diabetes in their lifetime; if both an individual's parents has Type 2 diabetes, their lifetime risk of developing the disease at some point rises to above 50 percent (Jarvis and Rubin, 2003). The trigger for all cases of Type 2 is that a lack of exercise and excess fat, impeding the action of insulin, meaning the body has an inability to cope with the metabolism of glucose.

Data now overwhelmingly suggests that sleep disruption also plays a major role in the development of Type 2 diabetes due to a pathway of adverse metabolic changes (Okada et al, 2006; Mallon et al, 2005; Punjabi et al, 2004; Ayas et al, 2003; Punjabi et al, 2002; Vgontzas et al, 2000). However, the increased risk of Type 2 diabetes and the contributory factor of reduced or continually interrupted sleep is not yet fully explored. A causal relationship between obesity and the onset of Type 2 diabetes (where insulin cannot function correctly in the presence of fat impeding its normal action on the cells) has long been established. However, a definitive link between a person having periods of reduced or interrupted sleep (so that they total less than eight hours per night) and that person going on to develop Type 2 diabetes as a result has not.

What is known is that a decrease in the amount of sleep per night increases obesity (Taheri et al, 2004; Cournot et al, 2004; Shigeta et al, 2001) which is a significant risk factor for the development of Type 2 diabetes. This increase in obesity is thought to be due to a reduction in energy expenditure during sleep and an alteration in the levels of the substances leptin and ghrelin when sleep is disturbed or lacking. Leptin is an appetite suppressant produced by adipose tissue and ghrelin is released by the stomach in response to fasting in order to promote the sensation of hunger (Gale et al, 2004). Studies have shown that the levels of leptin and ghrelin vary according to the amount and quality of sleep (Dzaja et al, 2004; Schoeller et al, 1997), with ghrelin levels dropping during the later stages of sleep as the individual goes without food, but rising again to cause a feeling of hunger in the morning.

Leptin levels, however, remain elevated throughout the night due to the influence of melatonin which enhances leptin production in the presence of insulin (Alonso-Vale, 2005). Melatonin is a hormone produced by the pineal gland, the action of which suppresses libido in accordance with the fight or flight response (as does the hormone cortisol) by reducing luteinizing hormone and follicle stimulating hormone secretion by the anterior pituitary gland. Whilst sleeping during the night hours, melatonin also enhances leptin level as an appetite suppressant hormone. This is because we do not need to induce a waking state in order to eat during normal sleeping hours, sleep being far more necessary for the brain and body cells. Increased levels of leptin (as an appetite suppressant) also reduces the action of ghrelin (making us hungry) preventing us from waking during the night due to hunger (Spiegel et al 2004a; Spiegel et al, 2004b). Thus, if sleep is disrupted, melatonin and leptin levels drop, ghrelin levels are raised, and appetite is not sufficiently suppressed so that the individual may decide to eat or drink at a time when they normally would not, increasing calorific intake.

Data therefore appears to suggest a strong association between reduced sleep or frequently disrupted sleep patterns and the development of

Type 2 diabetes over time due to metabolic disturbances increasing the body's glucose intolerance and insulin insensitivity (meaning that more insulin needs to be produced to lower blood glucose levels effectively). An increase in insulin insensitivity (a pre-cursor to the development of Type 2 diabetes) and insufficient beta cell compensation due to hormonal alterations has also been seen in people who work at night and sleep during the day (known as shift work disorder). Shift work, a necessary lifestyle for some people, changes the normal rhythmic patterns of melatonin release and this unnatural alteration means a raised level of melatonin is then present, inhibiting glucose-induced insulin release (the release of insulin by the beta cells in response to increased blood glucose levels) when the person eats or drinks so that blood glucose levels are higher than usual (Lyssenko et al, 2009).

During a normal period of eight hours' sleep food is not regarded as a priority whilst the body repairs itself. Therefore, if melatonin levels are adversely altered by a disruption in sleep patterns, appetite increases; the individual may eat more or need to eat at different times in the case of shift work, and insulin secretion in response to glucose is reduced. This is not the same as in Type 2 diabetes, where increased insulin is produced to try and lower blood glucose levels, because its action on cells is impeded by abnormal hormone levels. The result on blood glucose levels, however, is the same: blood glucose content is high and a diabetes-like state is reached.

## OBSTRUCTIVE SLEEP APNEA AND INSULIN LEVELS

Obstructive sleep apnea (OSA) is a condition causing intermittent and continual cessation of breathing leading to reduced levels of oxygen in the blood (Sharma and Kavuru, 2010). This condition is thought to be due to excess fat deposits around the neck area which compresses the trachea when an individual is horizontal during sleep, thus impeding movement and leading to snoring as air enters and leaves the constricted airway. A population-based survey carried out in the United States in

2005 showed that one in four adults were at risk from having OSA (Hiestand et al, 2006) and a further study showed that more than half of American adults who had been diagnosed with Type 2 diabetes also had OSA (Young et al, 2002).

An earlier correlation between diabetes, snoring and glucose intolerance was established in Britain (Norton and Dunn, 1985) and Europe (Jennum et al, 1993) for people with Type 2 diabetes caused by obesity, fat deposits around the neck inhibiting breathing and leading to snoring. The link between the development of Type 2 diabetes (due to obesity rather than hereditary factors) and snoring has also been established in a number of studies (Lindberg et al, 2007; Renko et al, 2005; Elmasry et al, 2000). It is clear that the underlying cause of both conditions is obesity, excess fat impeding the airways and the action of insulin upon the cells, increasing blood glucose levels because of the raised level of glucose adhering to the red blood cells, and increasing glucose intolerance, thus requiring the production of more insulin to deal with this.

Whilst it is true that not every person with obstructive sleep apnea is obese or has Type 2 diabetes, individuals who are not clinically obese but suffer from OSA have been found to have a higher level of fasting glucose and higher blood insulin levels (Vgontzas et al, 2000) suggesting a pre-diabetes state where excess glucose is not able to be cleared from the body, despite increased insulin secretion. Further investigation in this area has shown that mild obesity is also a pre-cursor to the development of impaired glucose tolerance (Punjabi et al, 2002) and insulin resistance (Ip et al, 2002). A marked improvement in insulin sensitivity (with a reduction in the amount of glucose adhering to red blood cells) has been seen with the use of continuous airway pressure therapy for obstructive sleep apnea for people with and without diabetes (Çuhadaroğlu et al, 2009; Dorokova et al, 2008; Brooks, 1994).

These results suggest that improving breathing and in turn improving sleep quality impact largely on metabolic function and insulin sensitivity (important in the regulation of increased blood glucose levels), although

Marks and Richmond (2007) state that a substantial and prolonged reduction in oxygen (hypoxia) leads to low blood glucose levels (hypoglycaemia) by interfering with the body's ability to produce glucose. It appears, therefore, that sleep apnea alone, with its characteristic marked reduction in oxygen supply, is not singularly a trigger for Type 2 diabetes. Factors such as body mass index and a reduced duration of quality sleep over time also contribute to a diabetic state due to disruption in glucose metabolism.

This has been demonstrated in two randomised controlled trials. In the first, patients with both impaired glucose tolerance and severe sleep apnea used continuous airway pressure therapy over a six-week period whilst another group used a placebo treatment, then the treatments were swapped. The studies showed no change in the participants' metabolic status (Coughlin et al, 2007). In the second study, one group of patients with Type 2 diabetes and sleep apnea received continuous airway pressure therapy for three months whilst another group received a placebo treatment. This research also showed no difference in glycaemic control or insulin resistance between the two groups (West et al, 2007). It is clear then that further research is necessary in the areas of sleep disruption, Type 2 diabetes, insulin levels, and obstructive sleep apnea before any definitive causal link can been made.

# Chapter Two

# The historical use of insulin in psychiatry

The hormone insulin, as mentioned earlier, was discovered in 1921 by researchers Frederick Banting and Charles Best in Toronto, Canada. It is produced by the pancreas in order to maintain the amount of glucose in the blood. If there is too much insulin present, either in Type 1 diabetes from injection or due to excess because of factors such as alcohol metabolism or other natural or abnormal phenomenon (Wilson, 2011), hypoglycaemia, also known as insulin shock, results. As glucose is the primary source of fuel for the brain and nervous system and the main energy source for all other body cells, a dramatic reduction in this fuel in the presence of excess insulin in the body causes symptoms such as irritability, headache, blurred vision, confusion, disorientation, tiredness, dizziness, shaking, muscle weakness, nausea, palpitations, rapid heart beat, tingling in the fingers and around the mouth, loss of consciousness, and even coma if the deficit in glucose is severe and sustained.

Normal (in people who do not suffer from diabetes) blood glucose levels are between 4.0–7.0mmol/L (72–126mg/dl American measurement), but in cases of extreme hypoglycaemia, where there is a significant excess of insulin, blood glucose levels fall dangerously low to below 2mmol/L (36mg/dl) and death can eventually occur if this glucose deficiency is not corrected after 12 hours or more because brain function is reduced and cannot be sustained (Marks and Richmond, 2007). The liver stores the simple sugars fructose (from fruit), galactose (from milk) and glucose as glycogen for conversion when the blood glucose level falls too low. Around 60 percent of the glucose contained in a meal passes through the liver and enters the bloodstream for use as fuel by the body cells and 40 percent is stored by the liver as glycogen. Only the liver has this function and is able to return glucose to the blood when hypoglycaemia occurs; it can also create glucose from energy stores when there is a need, such as during a period of fasting or vigorous exercise.

As previously seen, insulin is necessary to make glucose available for the cells to use as fuel. When there is too much insulin, the effects of hypoglycaemia are caused by the brain's reaction to a lack of glucose as it struggles to carry out normal function and the liver releases glucose as a corrective response. In the event that the amount of insulin present is excessive, and where glycogen stores in the liver are depleted, brain damage occurs. If there is a large amount of insulin working for several hours with no glucose to counteract this, permanent damage results after the blood glucose level has remained very low at 1.1mmol/L (20mg/dl) or less for five hours or more (Marks and Richmond, 2007). However, full recovery can occur if the patient's blood glucose levels are kept within normal range for several days following severe hypoglycaemia. Death from hypoglycaemia is usually due to raised inter-cranial pressure and multi-organ failure after prolonged coma, although it is rare, or this may occur more quickly if there is a rush of adrenaline in response to hypoglycaemia causing electrical disturbance to the heart (Marks and Richmond, 2007)

Hypoglycaemia, occurring in diabetes and non-diabetes, can often be mild and the symptoms may even go unnoticed apart from a headache, irritability and a feeling of hunger. For most individuals whose diabetes is managed with several measured doses of insulin each day, any episode of hypoglycaemia is mostly mild and is easily treated. However severe hypoglycaemia, most commonly associated with Type 1 diabetes, may lead to unconsciousness because the brain has insufficient glucose to work optimally and continue vital functions such as respiration. Insulin-induced hypoglycaemia is an acute condition which is also seen in drug addicts who inject insulin in order to experience the rush of adrenaline that accompanies low blood glucose levels. Self-administration of insulin leading to hypoglycaemia requiring medical attention is almost as frequent for those without legitimate access to insulin on prescription as it is for people using it to treat their diabetes (Marks and Richmond, 2007).

Following severe hypoglycaemia and unconsciousness for a period of half-an-hour or more, experienced by the author with Type 1 diabetes and requiring assistance from another person in order to regain consciousness, the following unpleasant symptoms occur:

- After initial sweating and feeling very hot, severe low blood glucose levels lead to a fall in core body temperature (hypothermia) and an inability to get warm.

- A single episode of severe hypoglycaemia leaves me with prolonged muscle weakness and confusion for several hours after coma due to temporary deprivation of glucose for fuel.

- An episode of severe hypoglycaemia (<2mmol/L or 36mg/dl) results in a prolonged bad headache for the rest of the day, sometimes for the following day as well.

- In response to depleted glucagon stores, extreme hunger is experienced and the liver then raises blood glucose to hyperglycaemic levels (Sonkson and Sonkson, 2000). This is followed by sickness with the rapid rise in blood glucose and difficulty in returning glucose levels to within the normal range for a number of hours.

- During insulin-induced coma, I experience fitting and resultant brain damage occurs (Asvoid et al, 2010; Bree et al, 2009; Austin and

Deary, 1999). Once this stage is reached, recovery is accompanied by complete loss of memory of events prior to the episode.

- Recovery from severe hypoglycaemia is accompanied by a heightened emotional response, for example, extreme gratitude to the person who injected glucagon to reverse the hypoglycaemic coma.

Insulin, in excess, is therefore a mind-altering drug.

## INSULIN SHOCK TREATMENT

For many years at the beginning of the 20th century there had been a desire to find an effective treatment for the challenging condition of schizophrenia, the term used to describe a severe personality disorder first used by Swiss psychiatrist, Eugene Bleulter in 1911. Today it is estimated that one percent of the population throughout the world suffers from schizophrenia (Lewis and Levitt, 2002). Using M.R.I. scans, scientists have determined that in the first year following the diagnosis of schizophrenia, five percent of the brain is destroyed and after five years this figure rises to 25 percent (Zou et al, 2008). The scans clearly show that this destruction sweeps forward from the hind brain towards the frontal lobe, the area responsible for reasoning and emotional response, eventually impairing these functions.

Schizophrenia is therefore now recognised to be a brain disease akin to Altzheimer's in its destructive capacity, rather than being a mental illness which leaves the brain structurally unchanged but periodically affecting the individual, as with depression. The most common symptoms of schizophrenia include hallucinations, delusions, blunted emotions, disordered thinking, and a withdrawal from reality (Frith and Johnstone, 2003; Burns, 1991). This search for an effective treatment that worked was especially urgent because the understanding of the origin of schizophrenia and its diagnosis was, and still remains, extremely contentious. People with schizophrenia have historically been grossly misunderstood and shunned by society. The symptoms of schizophrenia were noted in Ancient Egypt, China, Hindu, Greek and Roman civilisations and during medieval times, people suffering with personality disorders such as schizophrenia were thought to exhibit these extreme behaviour traits due, undoubtedly, to demonic possession (Holland, 1590). Centuries later, understanding of this very challenging condition and its causes was not much better, although psychiatric hospitals now existed in order to try and relieve the suffering endured, and there was no shortage of people with schizophrenia filling these asylums. One such mental institution in the United States was Worcester State Hospital in Massachusetts whose records demonstrate the huge extent of the problem. For the year spanning 1929–1930, 83 (20 percent) of the 414 patients were admitted for the first time with a diagnosis of dementia praecox schizophrenia. Re-admissions with schizophrenia numbered 36 (42 percent) of 86 patients and over one-fifth (21 percent) of those who had died in hospital had schizophrenia. Shockingly, half of these individuals had been hospitalized because of their condition for twenty years or more (Department of Mental Diseases, Annual Report of the Trustees of the Worcester State Hospital, 1930).

Depending on individual perspective, a particularly unfortunate decision for patients or a major contribution to psychiatric care was to treat the symptoms of addiction, psychosis and schizophrenia using insulin. Polish Austrian-American, Manfred Sakel, was a neuropsychiatrist working as an intern at the Lichternfelde Hospital for Mental Diseases, an addiction sanatorium frequented by the famous in Berlin (Alexander et al, 1966). Dr Sakel's experimentation began when he was treating a diabetic actress who was staying at the sanatorium because she was addicted to morphine and received treatment to attempt to break her addictive behaviour. Sakel, as her psychiatrist and also treating her diabetes during her stay, wrongly gave her too much insulin (he was clearly familiar with treating the mind but not the body) which plunged her into a hypoglycaemic coma. Although this was an unfortunate and potentially serious mistake, he found that the actresses' incessant cravings for her morphine addiction were much diminished following the hypoglycaemic coma, as was the excited state usually associated with morphine withdrawal. Therefore Sakel arrogantly pronounced that he had permanently cured her (Alexander et al, 1966).

Sakel felt, following this unexpected and accidental discovery, that this treatment had been so effective in reversing addictive symptoms in this one patient that he published his findings (Sakel, 1930). He then carried out numerous experiments and continued to perfect the use of "insulin coma treatment" in animal studies. After a period of time during which he clearly judged he had achieved numerous successful outcomes he applied the treatment to other human subjects. He was of the opinion that there was definite marked improvement in his patients' psychotic symptoms and began using insulin coma treatment in patients with other mental health conditions, such as anorexia, where the presence of a large amount of insulin in the body made the sufferer hungry. With such encouraging results he named his accidental discovery the "Sakel Technique": subduing patients with insulin coma and hypoglycaemic convulsions in order to diminish (mask) their severe symptoms of psychosis and schizophrenia.

Putting forward a rationale for the reason why the animals in his experiments and his patients exhibited less severe symptoms following insulin coma, Sakel reasoned that this was due to the way low blood glucose levels adversely affected brain function. He stated that because of the clear way the brain is disturbed in conditions such as addiction, psychosis and schizophrenia, it followed that inducing insulin shock (the effects of achieving very low blood glucose levels) may counter the symptoms of these conditions and calm the patient as brain function would eventually be strengthened by sustained and periodic deprivation of glucose. However, the brain cannot learn to do without glucose as it is required to maintain normal function. As mentioned previously, following his mistaken overdosing of the diabetic actress with insulin in 1927, Sakel introduced his Insulin Shock or Insulin Coma Treatment which he later justified:

My supposition was that some noxious agent weakened the resilience and the metabolism of the nerve cells ... a reduction in the energy spending of the cell, that is in invoking a minor or greater hibernation in it, by blocking the cell off with insulin will force it to conserve functional energy and store it to be available for the reinforcement of the cell (Sakel, 1930).

In 1933, Dr Sakel took his now renowned and well-practised treatment method to Vienna's University Neuropsychiatric Clinic, emphasising that he had personally witnessed a tremendous improvement rate in as many as 88 percent of his cases, this improvement being backed up by certain key studies (Whitaker, 2010; Valenstein, 1986). Quite worryingly, Slater and Sargeant (1944) later wrote that at the time of asylums learning to administer this new schizophrenia intervention, the insulin coma treatment technique could be learnt from books alone, although some practical experience was desirable to avoid the dangers of the procedure. From Vienna the use of insulin coma treatment quickly spread and from 1934, it was introduced to the United States where the idea was quickly taken on as it offered new hope in the treatment of chronic psychiatric disorders for thousands of people.

Sakel heavily emphasised the "shock" element of insulin coma treat-ment, believing that if the body was forced to deal with the shock of low blood glucose levels, lowered blood pressure, extreme sweating, and increased heart and respiration rates, the brain in turn could not fully focus on the symptoms of mental health conditions; therefore, these would diminish if not disappear completely as brain cells learnt to cope with more stress over time. Uptake of the new treatment in England was less speedy due to the intervention of World War 2 in 1939, although insulin coma treatment was used extensively at the Maudsley psychiatric hospital in London in the late 1930s. As previously seen, Sakel's miracle discovery was now used not only in treating addictive behaviours but also to address the debilitating symptoms of schizophrenia; an umbrella treatment covering all psychiatric conditions. His unique contribution to the field of psychiatric care was grasped enthusiastically by the numerous institutions trying to cope with the debilitating effect schizophrenia had on its patients as, at that time, they had little else to offer them.

Dr Sakel taught other physicians his perfected technique of gradually introducing the patient to what he called a small amount of insulin to achieve a semi-comatose state, but not as far as deep, unresponsive unconsciousness. The treatment technique widened in usage as doctors attended other institutions who had already adopted the idea of insulin shock treatment on a wide scale, these individuals learning from books and by observation, then taking the idea back to their own mental health establishments. These keen to learn physicians were instructed that patients undergoing insulin coma therapy should all be treated together in a large, warm room because severe hypoglycaemia leads to extreme sweating before hypothermia occurs (Wilson, 2011). Semi-conscious subjects had been known to throw the blankets off their beds and remove their clothes due to feeling so hot in the process of their blood glucose level falling dangerously low.

A team of experienced nursing staff with a psychiatrist allocated to each patient were present to administer the insulin and observe the dramatic mental and physical effects on these individuals in the hours that followed (Slater and Sargeant, 1944). The treatment began with an injection of up to 20 units of insulin early in the morning, an amount which a person with Type 1 diabetes might take for a large, carbohydrate-rich meal; only these individuals were not permitted to eat after their evening meal the night before. The treatment was doubled to 40 units of insulin on day two; 60 units on day three; 80 on day four; and 100 units on day five. On the sixth day the overall dosage was halved, and on the seventh day, the patient's bodies were permitted to rest before the gruelling regime recommenced again the following week for a period of six weeks in total. The insulin dosage was only increased by 20 units per day until unconsciousness was achieved, then the dosage remained stable; it was injected into muscle rather than into subcutaneous fat for a faster uptake.

The desired unconscious state could be quickly achieved in some patients with as little as 40 units of insulin per day to maintain a state of coma for three to four hours although in rare cases, the dose needed to be increased to a hefty 240 units (enough for eleven to twelve large, carbohydrate-rich meals for a person with Type 1 diabetes), followed on subsequent days by 40 units, then 240 units again to increase insulin sensitivity, although a dose as high as 600 units of insulin was reported as being used in one "difficult" patient (Slater and Sargeant, 1944; Sakel 1937a; 1937b). Whilst Slater and Sargeant (1944), and Manfred Sakel, stated that coma should be maintained for three to four hours, and personal accounts of undergoing insulin coma treatment also attest to this, the experience of other patients was a coma length of half-an-hour to an hour in duration. This suggests that each physician had his own methods and preferred coma length, and also that coma may not have been achieved as easily in some patients as others. Psychiatric patients who were young and lean would have succumbed to the effects of excess insulin very quickly.

A true understanding of the complexities of insulin sensitivity had only recently been achieved in 1935 when Sir Harold Himsworth, a diabetes specialist, discovered that the body is more sensitive to insulin when there is a low amount of body fat, as fat impairs the action of insulin. He experimented by giving people with Type 1 diabetes, who produce no insulin at all and are usually thin, glucose and insulin simultaneously. He also repeated the experiment in people with Type 2 diabetes, who produce a large amount of insulin in response to glucose but cannot utilise it as fuel because of a greater degree of body fat which impairs the ability of insulin to lower blood glucose. Himsworth discovered that those with Type 1 diabetes were insulin sensitive, where the insulin injected had worked on the glucose that was consumed so that the insulin and glucose effectively cancelled each other out, keeping the individual's blood glucose level stable. Conversely, he found that people with Type 2 diabetes were insulin insensitive; the insulin injected was not utilised to metabolise the glucose eaten because body fat impeded the use of insulin by the cells, causing the blood glucose level to rise to an abnormal level (Krentz and Himsworth, 2011; Himsworth, 2011). This research showed that the body's uptake of insulin is dependent on the level of insulin present and the degree of sensitivity to it. The insulin coma treated patient injected with the all-time record of 600 units of insulin was no doubt insulin insensitive (with excess body fat) if he/she did not succumb to unconsciousness with a much smaller insulin dose. We now know that it would take a dose of around 1,000 units of insulin to kill a person who is obese and insulin resistant, although a fatal dosage varies from person to person due to the amount of body fat; an individual would also have died during insulin coma treatment if their blood glucose level fell to less than 2mmol/L (36mg/dl) causing unconsciousness for a period of twelve hours or more (Marks and Richmond, 2007). The psychiatric objective of insulin coma treatment was to achieve unconsciousness for at least one hour and a maximum of four.

## COMPLICATIONS OF INSULIN COMA TREATMENT

In 1956, Manfred Sakel stated that in his opinion, over twenty-eight years of continual experience applied to a range of psychiatric problems, insulin coma treatment had established its absolute value beyond any possibility of doubt in the world of psychiatry (Sakel, 1956). From the mid-1960s, insulin coma treatment was gradually discontinued, perhaps because after thirty-seven years of subjecting patients to the grim and ultimately dangerous side-effects of severe hypoglycaemia it was finally realised that the barbaric treatment did not actually work because schizophrenia cannot be cured. It was also a very expensive treatment to administer on such as widespread basis as it required high staffing levels, many man-hours, and numerous trained psychiatrists, nursing staff and orderlies to be present (Alexander, 1966).

From the physician's perspective, anti-psychotic medications, such as Chlorpromazine (coincidentally a drug known to block the action of insulin and cause hyperglycaemia), to control and manage the symptoms of schizophrenia were much cheaper, did not present a treatment that was time-consuming to administer to patients, and was far more effective in controlling the symptoms of the condition. Although insulin coma treatment was no longer being prescribed for sectioned patients in psychiatric institutions, it was never actually officially banned. Because inducing severe hypoglycaemia in people with schizophrenia was felt to result in too many adverse reactions, it was gradually phased out of use by mental institutions around the world; the most adverse of these being death.

As mentioned previously, severe hypoglycaemia is very dangerous and damaging to the brain, resulting in lasting brain damage (Auer, 2004a; 2004b; Austin and Deary, 1999). Death from severe hypoglycaemia is fortunately rare among those with diabetes taking insulin or due to the malicious administration of insulin, due perhaps to the much smaller dosages than those used in insulin coma treatment. Death from hypogly- caemia is always preventable and reversible with the administration of intravenous glucose (Marks and Richmond, 2007). If death does occur it is usually due to raised inter-cranial pressure and multi-organ failure after prolonged coma, although this does not occur often. This may happen more quickly if there is a rush of adrenaline released into the bloodstream in response to very low blood glucose levels causing electrical disturbance to the heart (Marks and Richmond, 2007).

Death associated with insulin coma treatment however was not such a rare event, but doctors assessed the risks of death or brain damage from dangerously low and sustained blood glucose levels as being generally less of a concern than waiting for the spontaneous remission of schizo- phrenia (Slater and Sargeant, 1944). The same was said of the frequently lasting intellectual impairment that resulted from brain damage due to severe hypoglycaemic coma; that this was better for the patient than the disability caused by schizophrenia itself. Therefore, the need was seen as outweighing the risk. Mortality statistics collated in the United States for deaths occurring due to severe hypoglycaemia in insulin coma-treated patients numbered 90 people out of 12,000 (Slater and Sargeant, 1944). It is not clarified whether these deaths were a total amassed over the decade following Sakel introducing insulin coma treatment to the US in 1934 to the time that Slater and Sargeant were writing in 1944, or whether this figure was calculated as an average per annum. Nonetheless, if the former, 90 deaths over ten years gives a figure of nine patients with schizophrenia dying per year from the treatment they were given.

Half of these 90 deaths, as recorded on the individual's death certificate, were due to "hypoglycaemic encephalopathy", or disease of the brain brought about by very low blood glucose levels. Slater and Sargeant (1944) admitted that these deaths most frequently occurred when a patient had been under the supervision of psychiatrists (not medical doctors) with far less-experience in carrying out the treatment procedure. Therefore, they were negligent in allowing the patient to go too far into hypoglycaemic coma so that the brain struggled to keep vital functions going and fatal brain damage led to respiratory and cardiac arrest. Patients who eventually died of hypoglycaemic encephalopathy should have been treated immediately with intravenous glucose before the condition became irreversible, but inexperience with this procedure proved fatal.

Other causes of death during or following the administration of insulin coma treatment were given in state records as 12 fatalities from heart failure, probably brought about by a rush of adrenaline in response to severe hypoglycaemia putting the heart under extreme stress. Nine patients were recorded as having died from aspiration pneumonia, or inflammation of the lung tissue as a result of inhaling into the lungs infected material from the paranasal sinuses, from infected bronchi, or the inhalation of food or vomit (Loveday, 1991) whilst undergoing insulin coma treatment. Seven other people also died from pneumonia attributed to "other causes" such as following a chest infection.

Schizophrenia is a condition which leaves patients more susceptible to infection, perhaps because of lapses in personal care associated with the illness, or due to body shape. In 1925, a psychiatrist named Kretschmer noted that people who were institutionalised with schizophrenia tended to be tall and rather lean with angular faces (Burns, 1991). Of those with schizophrenia who died whilst undergoing insulin coma treatment, Slater and Sargeant (1944) suggested that this might be because the patients' build (slight) and general body health had rapidly deteriorated since the diagnosis of schizophrenia, leaving them far more susceptible to infections such as pulmonary tuberculosis, a condition which killed one further insulin coma patient.

Due to the severe reduction of glucose to the brain during frequent sessions of insulin coma treatment, many patients experienced extremely unpleasant epileptic-like fits which were precisely recorded as lasting for three-quarters of an hour up to one hour and forty minutes (Slater and Sargeant, 1944). Fits occurring during hypoglycaemic coma are very dangerous as they cause severe shock to the body and resultant brain damage, and it may take a longer period to reverse the hypoglycaemia with glucose than if fitting does not occur. Warren et al (2007) have shown that severe and recurrent hypoglycaemia results in varying degrees of subsequent learning impairment, a reduction in the ability to consolidate information and lapses in memory of short-term events. In cases where severe hypoglycaemia has led to protracted coma, Magnetic Resonance Imaging has shown that this results in permanent neurological dysfunction and structural abnormality of the brain, with the development of lesions in the frontal lobe and deep grey matter (Cranston, 2005).

Other imaging studies have confirmed that when hypoglycaemia is severe the brain goes into a state of shock with fitting occurring as a result; after the patient recovers there is long-term cognitive impairment and lasting damage to the brain's cortex and hippocampus regions (Bree et al, 2009). Marks and Richmond (2007) have also stated that when the brain is deprived of glucose during severe hypoglycaemia this is accompanied by seizures because the brain has insufficient glucose to function normally. Resulting brain damage following severe and frequent episodes of hypoglycaemia therefore appears to be a consistent finding.

There were certain selection criteria imposed as a guideline to the type of patients deemed unsuitable to undergo insulin coma treatment. Those with schizophrenia and other chronic health conditions such as advanced cardiac disease; Grave's disease (a type of goitre associated with an over-active thyroid gland); either Type 1 or Type 2 diabetes; and people with advanced liver and kidney disease that had resulted in a pronounced functional impairment were thought unsuitable for the therapy as these conditions contraindicated its use. However, Slater and Sargeant (1944) only suggested that treating people with these chronic illnesses "can be dangerous". With these conditions there could be a much greater chance of death during hypoglycaemia as there was more to go wrong, but the treatment was decided at the psychiatrist's discretion. People over the age of forty-five were also felt to be more of a mortality risk and were judged less likely to achieve remission from their schizophrenia as a result of insulin coma treatment. Perhaps this was a get-out clause put in place by physicians who were rapidly realising by the mid-1940s that insulin coma treatment did not bring about lasting effects or permanent remission.

Wootton (2006), in his brilliant book, *Bad Medicine: Doctors Doing Harm Since Hippocrates*, has stated that, according to the doctor treating the condition, the burden of responsibility concerning any failure of a medical treatment to bring about a cure lay with the patient themselves. This is because doctors specialise in certain diseases solely in order to alleviate their patient's symptoms as described to them by the sufferer, their overall concern being to make the individual feel better, if not in the short term, then in the longer term. In other words, if the prescribed treatment did not work, the doctor blamed the patient for not taking their medication or utilising their treatment regime as they were instructed. Perhaps then using extensive criteria to contraindicate insulin coma treatment in anyone over forty-five, or an individual with schizophrenia accompanied by another chronic health condition, allowed psychiatrists at the time to cite the lack of available treatments for these specific patients as a reason why so many individuals were incarcerated for decades in mental asylums.

## An equally shocking treatment

Another unfortunate and cruel treatment devised to treat patients with psychoses, designed to shock the brain and reduce the symptoms of schizophrenia, was to induce a controlled epileptic fit. Almost simultaneous with Manfred Sakel's discovery of insulin coma and its observed effects on a diabetic actress with morphine addiction, Ladislas von Meduna began clinical experiments on animal subjects in Hungary with the convulsant-inducing drug, Metrazol in 1933. Meduna, a Hungarian physician working at the Interacademic Institute of Psychiatric Research in Budapest, observed what he thought was a "biological antagonism" (meaning that one condition could not fully manifest its symptoms in the presence of another) in patients who suffered from both of the conditions of schizophrenia and epilepsy (Mackay, 1965).

As such, and seemingly with little knowledge of Sakel's work with insulin coma and schizophrenia patients, Meduna tested his hypothesis to develop the theory that artificially inducing an epileptic fit in an individual with schizophrenia would lead to a cure of the former condition as, in his opinion, having both epilepsy and schizophrenia effectively cancelled each other out. Meduna conducted various trials with the intra-muscular injection of several convulsion-inducing drugs to try and achieve the desired effect. Camphor was injected into human subjects, although it is poisonous in large quantities, the effect causing symptoms similar to those of hypoglycaemia: irritability, disorientation, muscle spasm, lethargy, convulsions and seizures (Pearce, 2008). Strychnine administered to patients in a large enough dosage caused their body to arch sharply backwards as the muscles in the back, going into agonising spasm, are stronger than the muscles in the chest. Thebain, an opiate and class A drug similar to morphine and codeine, caused convulsions and fits in the test subjects, but not in a way conducive to Meduna's idea of obliterating schizophrenic symptoms.

Pilocarpine, as a constituent of eye drops, causes the ciliary muscles in the eyes to contract (Rosin, 1991) but when injected as a large dose, compromises the blood-brain barrier, entering the brain and causing convulsions and fits. This drug was not only dangerous for this reason, but it did not result in predictable seizures. Sakel had also used combinations of these substances to enhance the effects of insulin coma (Sakel, 1937b). Meduna tested the effects of each drug on first animal, then human subjects in order to repeatedly achieve a controllable level of seizure; judged enough to shock the patient's brain out of its schizophrenic confines. Finally, Meduna experimented with Pentilenetetrazol, or Metrazol (Fink, 1985; 1984). Only Metrazol had the desired effect he was hoping to achieve: the rapid onset of convulsions after injection that were both varying in their severity according to dosage and which caused intense seizures.

Similar to Sakel, Meduna announced in 1937 that after using Metrazol treatment extensively in 110 of his resident schizophrenic patients, half were deemed so spectacularly recovered that they were able to be discharged from hospital and, like Sakel, Meduna even claimed that some were remarkably cured of their condition. Sakel clearly had competition for his insulin coma treatment and, not only that, Metrazol convulsion therapy was far more cost-effective, requiring fewer staff and man hours to administer and manage the after effects. However, Metrazol was far more potent than insulin in its affect on the patient which could not simply be reversed with glucose when things suddenly got out of control. An added negative point for patients was that the convulsions induced were so severe that they resulted in spinal fractures (due to the similar effects of extreme muscle spasms in the back seen in strychnine poisoning), lung abscesses and pneumonia (Beckenstein, 1939).

Two years later in 1939 the scientific community regarded Meduna's theory of "biological antagonism" in patients with schizophrenia and epilepsy as ridiculous and Metrazol therapy as highly dangerous; Metrazol was, however, effective in treating both manic and psychotic depression and was used up until the late 1940s. This paradigm shift in thinking made insulin coma therapy appear the far more favourable option as a treatment choice, and this was confirmed in controlled research trials (Stephens et al, 2000; Fink, 1985) comparing the effects of insulin coma treatment and Metrazol. As mentioned earlier, insulin coma therapy continued to be used until it was gradually phased out in the 1960s when more effective schizophrenia medications, such as Chlorpromazine, became widely available.

## THE PATIENT'S PERSPECTIVE OF INSULIN COMA THERAPY

There are several harrowing accounts available of the patient's experience of repeatedly undergoing and surviving insulin coma treatment. Perhaps the most well-known of these is that of Dr John Nash; his experience, schizophrenia, and continued battle to maintain his mathematical genius portrayed in the book, *A Beautiful Mind* (Nasar, 1998), which was later made into a film in 2002. Nash is a brilliant Senior Research Mathematician and economist at Princeton University working in the field of game theory: how chance governs the systems used in daily life (Nash, 2007). He shared a Nobel Memorial Prize in Economic Sciences in 1994 with game theorists Reinhard Selten and John Harsanvi. Nash had formerly been a mathematics instructor from 1951 at the Massachusetts Institute of Technology, where he met his wife, Alicia Lopez-Harrison de Lardé whom he married in February 1957.

In early 1959 Nash first recognised that his illness was becoming increasingly disruptive to his work; his wife was also pregnant at the time. Nash had developed disturbing symptoms of schizophrenia: paranoia, erratic behaviour, talking of people who were a danger to him (men wearing red ties who were part of a communist conspiracy to harm him), and seeing encrypted messages in newspaper articles (Nasar, 1998), the frequency of which completely overshadowed his academic work. As a result of Nash's disturbing symptoms, in April 1959 his wife took the very difficult and brave step of committing him to the McLean psychiatric hospital in Boston, a major teaching and research institution affiliated with Harvard Medical School. There he was diagnosed with paranoid schizophrenia due to his auditory disturbances and altered perceptions, lack of motivation and depression (Nasar, 1998).

Nash received injections of the anti-psychotic drug Chlorpromazine, psychotherapy and counselling treatment. He was released after six weeks but was not fit enough to return to teaching as his chronic psychosis remained uncured. Nash therefore resigned his teaching post and pension at M.I.T and the talented scientist left to seek political asylum in Europe for two years, first in France and then Germany. After facing increasing difficulties coping with the effects of his illness in Paris then Geneva, he was arrested and deported back to America at the request of the US government (Nasar, 1998). Despite Nash still being caught in the vice of failing mental health, well-meaning friends encouraged him to take up teaching once again in the hope that the regular routine of working would help ease his symptoms. Dr Nash, by reputation, then secured a position at Princeton University in 1961 where he remained for a year before he went back into hospital, residing there periodically over the next nine years.

Inevitably, with no available and effective medication to manage the condition, he was unable to win the battle of controlling the symptoms of his schizophrenia which worsened to a point that forced him back into a state hospital to request further treatment. As previous treatment with Chlorpromazine and group and individual talking therapies had failed to rid Nash of his schizophrenic symptoms, the condition which had lain dormant once again re-emerged. The majority of suitable treatment options had already been exhausted by the psychiatrists responsible for Nash's care. In the case of electro-convulsive therapy (E.C.T.), Dr Nash rationalised that it would undoubtedly affect his memory, reasoning and ability to ponder and address essential issues in the course of his work. These cognitive disturbances, in addition to restricting his movements and thought processes, would affect his speech as if he had suffered a stroke, and impair his ability to read or study, either for research or pleasure, his own work or the work of others.

Electro-convulsive therapy was introduced by the Italian neurologist, Ugo Cerletti in 1937. He had found that electric shock applied directly to the head of animals in his epilepsy research resulted in convulsions, and Cerletti knew that this also had an anaesthetic effect, having seen pigs prepared for slaughter in a similar way (Endler, 1988). Perfecting the technique on animals, Cerletti began to use the technique on human patients with severe schizophrenic symptoms, administering a series of ten to twenty electric shocks to the head on alternate days which he claimed resulted in the improvement of schizophrenic symptoms in most patients. In addition, a fortunate side-effect of the treatment was retrograde amnesia, meaning that patients could not remember the shocking experience or any subjective feelings about having electro convulsive therapy prior to the treatment.

In 1939, E.C.T. shock therapy had been extensively advertised and was in use widely in the Netherlands, France, Switzerland, England and the United States. However by the 1960s, its popularity had dramatically waned due to the availability of other less barbaric treatments, and a strong anti-E.C.T. lobby (Abrams, 1988) of the opinion that human beings should not be subjected to the cruelty of repeated electric shock to the head, a technique used to slaughter animals, and resulting in the distinct adverse after-effects on the personality and cognitive ability. Not surprisingly, Dr John Forbes Nash declined to undergo E.C.T. treatment, as to agree and suffer memory loss and impairment of his cognitive ability in this way would have been unbearable. This does, however, imply that other patients forcibly committed to mental health establishments did have the opportunity to make an informed choice regarding their treatment options and were therefore empowered, although this might not have been the case for every patient; Dr Nash being an exception because of his renowned brilliance.

A far worse and more permanent treatment option, if not choice for patients with schizophrenia, was to undergo a frontal lobotomy which would have rendered the talented academic permanently devoid of his personality and emotions. A frontal lobotomy is defined as psychosurgery; "the selective surgical removal of destructive nerve pathways or normal brain tissue with a view to influencing behaviour" (Gostin, 1980; Bridges and Bartlett, 1977; Barraclough and Mitchell-Heggs, 1974). This procedure involved surgically severing the connections between the prefrontal cortex and underlying structures of the brain, or completely destroying the frontal cortex tissue in the hope that this would release the emotional and intellectual areas of the brain. In an article written in 1942, the authors cited the drastic surgery as highly successful in reversing persistent aggressiveness, combativeness, and destructiveness, and that the procedure brought significant improvement warranting further investigation regarding its use in psychiatric disturbance (Cohen et al, 1942). This procedure fortunately eventually became outmoded with the growing use of anti-psychotic medication, although lobotomies were still carried out in the US, Britain and Scandinavia well into the 1980s (Valenstein, 1986).

Insulin coma treatment remained as a viable alternative, although many hospitals had turned against the once-popular miracle cure introduced by Dr Manfred Sakel as its effects, as well as being barbaric, were not permanent and frequently resulted in lasting brain damage to the patient. Insulin coma treatment was so popular that it had been used on a widespread basis in twenty-two different countries in the mid-1930s, and in the USA in the mid-1940s, insulin coma treatment was one of the three leading therapies used for patients diagnosed with schizophrenia, along with E.C.T. and drug medication. Insulin coma treatment was used so frequently in the desperate hope of offering a cure or respite to patients with psychiatric illness that in America alone, 75,000 people had received the treatment between 1935 and 1941 (Valenstein, 1986).

Manfred Sakel had reported that following several weeks of treatment, patients showed a continuing interest in their personal appearance and current events; markedly increased socialisation, having meals in the dining room with other residents rather than in their rooms in isolation; a blossoming personality and the ability to develop a number of new friendships with other patients to the extent that the patient's personality was unrecognisable as that of the original person (Sakel, 1937a). Adding credence to the success of the popular treatment were two large and supportive scientific studies which stated positive findings. In the first conducted by Ross and Malzberg in 1939, of 1,757 patients diagnosed with schizophrenia undergoing insulin coma treatment, 193 were judged to be permanently cured; 466 patients were thought to be very much improved; and a further 466 showed some improvement following their treatment. It is not noted whether these findings were statistically significant and the measure of improvement is questionable as it appears to have been based on subjective opinion. Despite this research and a further study in 1942 carried out at Pennsylvania State hospital, longitudinal evidence proved that any change was somewhat transitory and insulin coma treatment did not result in any lasting cure for schizophrenia.

The effect of depleting glucose as the brain's primary fuel source was not a permanent state, as well as being highly dangerous. Many physicians soon grew to realise this and felt that anti-psychotic medication was a preferred treatment alternative which, whilst not able to cure the patient, could in many cases subdue and bring under control the dramatic symptoms. Later evidence-based studies supported the opinion that insulin coma treatment was not a suitable or effective option for people with schizophrenia (Whitaker, 2010; Lifshutz, 1954). In 1961 at the time of Dr John Forbes Nash's continuing illness, Trenton State hospital in New Jersey still used insulin coma therapy as a treatment option for schizophrenia.

The remaining treatment options for Dr Nash were limited, and he was perhaps encouraged to try insulin coma treatment because his colleagues at Princeton University had advocated its use, possibly because its effects on the brain were less drastic than surgically removing the frontal lobe. However as an alternative, the thought of voluntarily agreeing to undergo numerous episodes of severe hypoglycaemia as a last resort is, to the author as an academic and diabetic, a courageous, thought-provoking and eternally hopeful decision because the effects of depleted glucose levels on the body are very frightening and distressing. Thoughts rush through the brain which appear extremely profound; however, there is no way to communicate them to others as spoken or written sentences are garbled and listeners assess the ramblings as that of a drunk.

Even for those who know that speech and brain activity are severely impaired by very low blood glucose levels, any attempt by the sufferer at communication is dismissed as rubbish, not making sense because of hypoglycaemia, or due to the person's distress at their condition. I can only deduce that Dr John Nash would have felt much the same, although doomed to endure hypoglycaemia for hours rather than it being quickly treated with glucose for diabetic hypoglycaemia. It is even more poignant that Nash was not helped by any of the available treatment options for schizophrenia as there is no cure, only management of the condition; none of which were effective for his brilliant mind.

John Nash's experience of insulin coma treatment at Trenton State hospital began when he was woken at six in the morning and denied breakfast, which would have raised his blood glucose levels and been counter-productive to insulin coma treatment, then dressed in cotton clothing to allow his skin to breathe whilst he sweated profusely as a consequence of the effects of too much insulin (Wilson, 2011). Nash was taken to a large room designated for insulin coma treatment, shared with a number of other patients undergoing the same fate, where he was assigned a metal bed with side rails to restrain and prevent falling out and injury when and if convulsions occurred. A nurse took his temperature, measured his blood pressure and heart rate; each of these changing drastically with severe low blood glucose levels, then the assigned dose of insulin was injected into either the shoulder or buttock muscle (Slater and Sargeant, 1944).

The types of insulin available and suitable for inducing coma in patients within a short space of time were either quick-acting soluble or fast-acting regular insulin (Marwood, 1973).There were around fifty other patients also undergoing insulin coma treatment simultaneously, with the attendance of two or three psychiatrists, four nurses, and several assistants. The clinical white scene, with screaming, fitting or convulsing people lined up and restrained in beds, with nurses, orderlies and psychiatrists peering at them and taking notes, is akin to something from science fiction. It is difficult to comprehend how this must have felt for the patient; one imagines that the setting only added to their feelings of despair, fear and hopelessness.

The fast-acting insulin injected took around twenty minutes to half an hour to take effect if administered subcutaneously into the fat layer beneath the skin, but faster still if injected into muscle, or much more quickly and accurately if delivered into a vein, working on the level of blood glucose and bringing it down from a normal 4.0–7.0mmol/L (72–126mg/dl) to a hypoglycaemic state of <3mmol/L or lower (<54mg/dl). At this stage, John Nash was still conscious, but now very tired, experiencing the early symptoms of hypoglycaemia: confusion, disorientation, headache, and irritability as his brain was starved of glucose, profuse sweating, goose bumps, then feeling very cold, having a lack of muscle strength, a rapid heartbeat, tingling around the mouth and increased salivation.

Other patients did not always experience the profuse sweating but swiftly fell into a deeper hypoglycaemic state before their eventual unconsciousness where their major muscles twitched through lack of glucose, their skin being hot and dry. The insulin given to Nash was still working for several hours and, over the following fifteen minutes, the remaining glucose in his blood was so depleted that there was little available for the insulin to act upon. As hypoglycaemic coma approached for the inmates, the muscles of the patient's arms and legs would jerk more violently and they showed symptoms akin to a grand mal epileptic fit 45 to 100 minutes after insulin was injected (Slater and Sargeant, 1944). When an individual shouted out and became a danger to themselves, they were restrained with a bed sheet pulled tightly over their body and then secured under the mattress to prevent injury to flailing limbs on the metal bed frame and side bars.

An hour to an hour and a half after the insulin was administered Nash was by now non-responsive to stimuli such as touch and sound. To test for the level of brain function at this stage, the patient's physician performed the Babinski reflex test. This reflex usually occurs in response to stroking the outer margin of the sole of the foot, where the big toe will move downwards if there is no neurological impairment and upwards if there is impairment present (Tortora and Grabowski, 1993). This is known as a stage-1 comatose state and the test was used in insulin coma treated patients to ascertain the level of unconsciousness achieved. As blood glucose levels were failing to rise sufficiently and naturally in the presence of a substantial insulin dose, the body would be struggling to rectify this imbalance as the liver released glucagon, adrenaline, noradrenaline, cortisol, growth hormone and vasopressin to increase the amount of glucose available to the brain (Marks and Richmond, 2007).

In the case of repeated insulin coma treatments, the patient's liver may have no longer had sufficient levels of stored glucose to release for this function; and with the amount of insulin being given with no food, the insulin outweighed the available glucose, sending the individual into a deeper stage 2 or stage 3 coma. As this occurred, the patient's breathing would become laboured as their brain fought to keep normal respiration and heart function going. The patient's closed eyes would have darted about, although a doctor checking the response of the pupils to light would have found that this reflex still functioned at this stage. Without available glucose though, the individual's larger muscles would have gone into spasm, with sweating remaining profuse as their temperature dramatically increased. As the coma deepened, the assigned doctor would have carried out further tests to assess the stage of hypoglycaemia. The physician would find the patient's pulse was fast and irregular, the reflexes of the corneas and the pupils to light were no longer present, and the deep tendon knee-jerk reflexes were lost.

The doctors and nursing staff present diligently checked all their comatose patients regularly in this way to assess their state every ten minutes; the patient was brought out of the coma with glucose thirty to sixty minutes after stage 2 coma was reached. The patient was revived with 200-300cc of 50 percent glucose solution administered via a naso-gastric tube, inserted into the nose and passing into the stomach. The glucose was quickly absorbed by the stomach lining, bringing the individual back to consciousness after several minutes. A further method of quickly introducing glucose to the body was to inject 25-50cc of 10 percent glucose solution intravenously; if patients awoke spontaneously because of the body's natural response to low blood glucose levels, sugared tea was given and patients were able to drink it themselves (Slater and Sargeant, 1944).

On regaining consciousness, the patient remained mentally and phys-ically slow for some fifteen minutes or more, their movement jerky, their speech slurred. As the recollection of their surroundings and situation returned, the patient would recognise a raging hunger as their liver craved an urgent source of glucose to replenish its depleted stores. The sweat-drenched bedclothes and cotton garments worn would be uncom-fortable and a nurse would accompany the individual to the showers for a wash and change before getting some longed-for breakfast. It is the author's experience that when eating following severe hypoglycaemia, excessive amounts are consumed because the brain is attempting to protect itself from a further lack of glucose. Patients treated with insulin coma treatment over a six week period showed considerable weight gain at the end due to this phenomenon (Slater and Sargeant, 1944).

This counter-regulation mechanism for glucose causes problems in the case of Type 1 diabetes because the blood glucose level then swings erratically upwards due to the hormones released and the food eaten. It is extremely difficult to exert self-control and only eat a measured amount of carbohydrates following severe hypoglycaemia; the hormonal imbalance alone can raise the blood glucose level to >18mmol/L (above

324mg/dl). Nash however, as a non-diabetic, would not have experienced this problem when trying to sate his hunger.

The overall aim of insulin coma treatment was to achieve a reduction in the patient's anxiety and psychotic symptoms (Sakel, 1937b). The success of the treatment had been widely acclaimed: increased calm, friendliness and sociability, fewer or even complete disappearance of hallucinations, and a reduction in anxious feelings, excitable episodes and the need for restraint. However, the signs were apparent that the brain had been irreparably damaged by repeated episodes of severe hypoglycaemic coma. Patients were more subdued, exhibited heightened emotions such as laughing or crying for no reason, had limb weakness, experienced errors when speaking (aphasia), and memory deficits. These changes have been shown to be due to death of sections of the brain. Animal studies have demonstrated that after 30–60 minutes of a very low blood glucose level of between 0.12 and 1.36mmol/L (2 and 24mg/dl) neuronal necrosis occurs, ultimately leading to a flat E.E.G. (electro encephalograph) reading (Auer, 2004a; 2004b).

In humans, the brain's cortex, basal ganglia and hippocampus are the most susceptible to sustained low blood glucose levels. Autopsies of those who have died after prolonged hypoglycaemia show widely distributed death of brain matter in the cerebral cortex (Bree, 2008; Comi, 1997; Patrick and Campbell, 1990). Conversely, a further study of geriatric patients with schizophrenia who had spent many years in mental asylums found that there was no notable cognitive decline between patients who had undergone insulin coma treatment and those who had not (Stephens et al, 2000). Those patients that survived the experience of insulin coma treatment were discharged back to their usual lives, continuing their treatment with drug medication and sessions of electro-convulsive therapy. Unfortunately for Dr Nash however, he returned to work after three years but inevitably succumbed to a relapse. Nash later admitted that he only took prescribed medication under pressure; after 1970 he was never committed to a psychiatric hospital again and refused any anti-psychotic drugs, his colleagues and students at Princeton Fine Hall mathematics centre accepting his eccentricities. From 2011 Nash's work has focused on advanced game theory.

A further personal recollection of undergoing insulin shock or coma treatment was given by Don Weitz in his account: *Insulin Shock - A Survivor's Guide to Psychiatric Torture* (2004). His experience of being involuntarily committed to the same institution as Nash, the McLean psychiatric hospital in Boston, began eight years earlier in 1951. Weitz, who was twenty years old at the time, stated that the reason his family had instigated this extreme intervention was due to a diagnosis of schizophrenia; a psychiatrist at McLean then advocating his suitability for insulin coma treatment or electric convulsive therapy (E.C.T.) on admission. This was no doubt due to his young age and physical, if not mental, fitness meaning he was judged as able to endure such a demanding treatment regime.

Although Don Weitz did not have to undergo E.C.T., seven weeks after being committed to the McLean mental institution he was subjected to the horror of insulin coma treatment. There was no explanation given to Weitz as a patient regarding what the procedure entailed, the likely and horrendous side effects or the risks involved when large and repeated doses of insulin are given to a human being. With no choice in the matter, Don Weitz was gradually introduced to 5 units of insulin per day until by day three, 25–30 units were being administered three times a day. This unnatural lowering of blood glucose levels had the effect of eliciting the usual side effects of profuse sweating, ravenous and unbearable hunger as the body tries to boost its glucose reserves, headaches, confusion, trembling, disorientation, muscle weakness and thrashing around in the confines of the metal bed in the treatment room. Due to his extreme hunger, the need for his body to replace glucose stores, and his body's defence mechanism to prevent this kind of ongoing depletion, Don Weitz ate ravenously after his coma sessions, gaining 49 pounds in weight as a result when the treatment had finished six weeks later.

It is a horrible feeling to find your vision blurred; your limbs shaking and weak; a growing feeling of panic bubbling inside your chest and complete disorientation as you rapidly lose control of your functions, unable to explain to those around you the enormity and urgency of the situation. For Weitz, undergoing this frightening effect not as an acute side effect of taking insulin to control diabetes, but because he was being forced to do so as a treatment that was supposedly doing him good, the repeated and seemingly unceasing phenomenon of severe hypoglycaemia must have been one hundred times worse.

In Don Weitz's emotionally resonant account of undergoing insulin coma treatment, he has managed to achieve something very poignant in recounting exactly how the experience of severe and repeated hypoglycaemia felt. Weitz has stated that on one disastrous occasion, he went much further than usual into a deeply unconscious state due to too much insulin being administered by the psychiatrist looking after him. As the aim of the treatment prescribed to Weitz was to keep patients in a subcomatose state rather than to induce a deep coma, this was clearly a dangerous mistake in insulin dosage and, Weitz reported that this fact was omitted purposely from his records which he was later permitted to see. He nonetheless had to endure the terrifying and amplified effects of deep hypoglycaemic coma, which he described as "debilitating and torturous"; a sentiment the author can wholeheartedly attest to.

Although it is barbaric to think that this "treatment" was designed to do good for people suffering from schizophrenia fortunately, as Weitz stated, the hypoglycaemic events, each lasting three to four hours in his case, could usually be rapidly reversed by drinking fruit juice with added glucose. This implies that the deep coma achieved by the doctor in charge of Weitz was indeed a mistake and that for the other episodes of hypoglycaemia he remained semi-conscious. However, whilst the effects were marginally less severe, being awake meant enduring the panic and fear induced by the treatment rather than being oblivious to it when unconscious.

Weitz recounted some of the unpleasant reactions he had to his prescribed treatment, noted by the nurses observing him. After 75 units of insulin he vehemently protested in his hypoglycaemic state that he could not possibly endure the treatment any longer; on another occasion he pleaded desperately that the treatment be discontinued and ravenously consumed a huge amount of food (implying food was available and patients could eat if they wished) to take up the insulin, raising his blood glucose levels against medical advice. On 90 units of insulin three times a day Weitz succumbed to a much deeper coma and thrashed around in an epileptic fit-like state, being non-responsive and not remembering the episode after medical staff brought him out of the coma with glucose.

The notes made by medical staff about Don Weitz frequently stated that he asked for the treatment to cease, and that on occasions he was unaware of what had happened to him, becoming highly emotional. From the author's perspective, if I am suffering a severe episode of hypoglycaemia and cannot help myself, I know that I am lucky enough to have someone else available doing all they can to help me reverse this state quickly. For Don Weitz, enclosed in a cool white and impersonal hospital room with up to fifty other patients lined up in rows on their metal beds and thrashing about or calling out with severe hypoglycaemia, induced by doctors supposedly for their own good, there was no one rushing to reverse the effect with the panacea of glucagon, sweet tea and calming words.

In total, Weitz endured 110 episodes of insulin-induced hypoglycaemia, emerging from the McLean psychiatric facility as a broken and shattered individual in 1953 at the age of twenty-two, a year after his insulin coma treatment ended. He stated that this was only due to his own ability to convince the McLean psychiatric staff that he was so much better for the experience; he would go back to university and undergo psychotherapy as an outpatient to control his condition, remaining well and out of hospital. One wonders the fate of those without the mental faculties to be empowered in this way? Bravely Weitz confronted his torturer after his release and asked why he had been subjected to insulin coma treatment, bearing in mind that an earlier course of psychotherapy would have been a far safer, cheaper and easier option for both patient and staff. His doctor patronised him, telling him his emotional reaction to being subjected to repeated induced hypoglycaemia was actually as a result of his illness, absolutely not because of the terrible nightmare he had experienced whilst in this psychiatrist's care.

It was the doctor's opinion that insulin coma treatment would be good for Weitz's "temper tantrums"; hardly surprising given that he had been forcibly committed to an institution by his family and had been subjected to the most horrific and barbaric experience that must have seemed endless. It is questionable whether doctors of the mind should have been allowed to instigate the injection of psychiatric patients with insulin when they sometimes did not have personal experience of the dangerous consequences. After all, Manfred Sakel himself only "discovered" insulin coma treatment in 1926 because he made a mistake with insulin dosage when injecting an actress who had diabetes, something that perhaps a trained nurse should have been doing at the hospital instead of a neuropsychiatrist, an error which would today ultimately result in a medical negligence or malpractice case. One wonders if Manfred Sakel, the instigator of this treatment method, or any of his followers, ever voluntarily underwent just one injection with a huge dose of insulin so that they could personally experience the terrifying and torturous effects of insulin overdose first hand? The answer is that this is highly unlikely.

> Men will always be mad and those who try to cure them are the maddest of all.
>
> Voltaire

# CHAPTER THREE

# INSULIN AS A PERFORMANCE-ENHANCING DRUG IN SPORT

Because insulin is thought to be an untraceable substance as it is naturally produced by the beta cells of the pancreas in non-diabetic individuals, opportunities to exploit its properties are many. One such area of insulin misuse, especially in recent times, is as a performance-enhancing drug in sport. Insulin can act as a powerful anabolic agent (creating larger molecules from smaller ones), to build muscle, increase strength and endurance for amateur and professional sportsmen and women. The use of performance-enhancing drugs by individuals to boost their sporting prowess is well-publicised in the media, and in many cases, more than one substance is abused in combination to increase muscle size, power and ability over others. Incidences of athletes doping themselves with substances to increase sporting performance, driven by a desire to be better than their competitors, reportedly goes back as far as the original Olympic Games (records kept from 776 BC).

Perhaps the most well known case of doping by an elite athlete in recent years is that of Lance Armstrong, who won numerous medals and titles in cycling. After long-term use of anabolic steroids, blood transfusions and blood boosters to carry more oxygen, he was revealed as a drug cheat and stripped of his seven Tour de France winning titles in 2012. He admitted to using a substance known as EPO (erythropoietin) which increases the production of red blood cells and therefore increases the body's oxygen-carrying capacity. This medication is intended to help people being treated with chemotherapy or who have chronic kidney failure and an impaired oxygen uptake by the red blood cells. A further well-profiled case of an athlete using drugs to win is that of Ben Johnson, the world class athlete who achieved two world records for the 100 metre sprint. Johnson was stripped of the gold medal he won at the Seoul Olympics in 1988 after he tested positive for anabolic steroid use and also admitted to the injection of growth hormone over many years (Moore, 2013).

The use of anabolic steroid substances in sport is widespread and in a study by Tricker et al (1989) it was shown that 54 percent of male and 10 percent of female bodybuilders admitted to having used steroids regularly. In a further study by Rich et al (1998) it was revealed that, in the United States alone, over one million elite and amateur athletes admitted that they had used performance-enhancing drugs. In addition, an estimated one-quarter of anabolic androgenic steroid use, such as testosterone, (responsible for the development of the sexual organs and secondary sexual characteristics in males), also included insulin because of its anabolic properties. Anabolic androgenic steroids are produced from derivatives of testosterone, the male hormone produced in the testes from puberty in males, although females typically also produce around 10 percent of the level seen in males (Tortora and Grabowski, 1993).

The use of anabolic steroid substances was perceived by abusers to be a necessary factor in order to win competitions with the added advantage of significantly increasing strength despite the known dangerous side-effects. The list of banned substances in sport, produced annually by the International Olympics Committee Medical Commission and Sub-Commission, is continually growing as the search by athletes goes on to find a drug that has the desired enhancement effect but also leaves the body very quickly, or is completely untraceable. For this reason, insulin, in combination with growth hormone and insulin-like growth factor-1, has become increasingly popular in the sporting world with non-diabetic athletes. As a result insulin was added to the list of banned substances for use in sport in 1998, the same year in which insulin became a prescription-only drug to prevent athletes buying the hormone from pharmacies. However, the determination of athletes to win at all costs means this in no barrier to obtaining banned substances such as insulin, especially now with their "no questions asked" availability on the Internet.

## THE EFFECT OF INSULIN AND OTHER HORMONES ON MUSCLE

There are a number of hormones used frequently by athletes, body builders, weight lifters and power lifters to build muscle, increase strength and endurance, and some of these hormones work in conjunction with one another to produce this desired effect. Growth hormone is a substance produced by the anterior pituitary gland, the amount of which is controlled by growth hormone releasing hormone and growth hormone inhibiting hormone (Tortora and Grabowski, 1993). The hormone is released in bursts during the early hours of sleep, during exercise, and at times of stress, reaching a maximum in the later teenage years and then steadily declining thereafter. Low blood glucose levels (when there is an excess of insulin or insufficient glucagon stored in the liver) encourage the release of growth hormone inhibiting hormone, which then in turn stimulates the production of human growth hormone to raise blood glucose levels. Once the blood glucose level returns to within normal range, growth hormone inhibiting hormone is released to prevent blood glucose levels rising too far. If hyperglycaemia occurs, this inhibits human growth hormone secretion and stimulates the secretion of growth hormone inhibiting hormone once more to reduce blood glucose levels.

It can be seen then that this is a very delicate balance, although manipulation by sports persons with additional injections of growth hormone and insulin can drastically alter both anabolism (the production of larger molecules from smaller ones) and catabolism (chemical reactions that break down complex organic compounds into simple ones with the release of energy) in the body. Growth hormone is a protein, like insulin, and therefore cannot be taken orally by athletes as it would be broken down into its component parts of amino acids and digested. As mentioned earlier with insulin, growth hormone is cleared from the body in the same way: by degradation in the liver and kidneys where it is passed out of the body in the urine. This means that only a very small amount of growth hormone remains in the urine, making it very difficult for doping authorities to test this in abusing athletes.

Growth hormone helps regulate many metabolic processes in the cells of the body, including the production of insulin-like growth hormone-1. This hormone is produced in the liver; the cells of mature cartilage, (known as chondrocytes) stimulating growth; in skeletal muscle fibres; connective tissue fibres (called fibroblasts); and other body cells. It was originally thought that insulin-like growth factor-1 was responsible and therefore necessary for many of the actions of growth hormone, although it is now considered that insulin-like growth factor-1 acts as an indicator for the action of growth hormone on the liver (Sonksen, 2001). In turn, insulin-like growth factor-1 is not regulated solely by growth hormone itself, but majorly by the level of nutrition and thyroid hormones present in the bloodstream (Tortora and Grabowski, 1993).

In order to work correctly, insulin-like growth factor-1 injection by athletes also requires a high carbohydrate and high protein diet for cellular reproduction to occur (Rashid et al, 2007). This is demonstrated when there is poor nutrition and in cases of undiagnosed or poorly managed Type 1 diabetes, where these states are associated with low plasma levels of insulin-like growth factor-1 and increased levels of growth factor (Sonksen, 2001). Although both growth hormone and insulin-like growth factor-1 have their own roles in the human body, they do work in conjunction with one another in a complex process that is not yet fully understood. Because some of the main functions of growth hormone are to regulate protein synthesis and mobilise fat (via a process known as lipolysis), this hormone is of great benefit to athletes and can be manipulated by those wishing to cheat the system. These two actions convert dietary calories solely into protein and therefore, muscle. Insulin-like growth factor-1 also stimulates protein synthesis in this way, but not as robustly as growth hormone (Sonksen, 2001). Insulin has the effect of preventing protein breakdown, so that, taken together, growth hormone, insulin-like growth factor-1 and insulin allow new muscle to be formed and not broken down again.

Since the early 1980s, growth hormone has been abused by athletes to alter anabolism and muscle composition as it has a peak action period of 1–3 hours and is undetectable after 24 hours (Sonksen, 2001). The potential of insulin to have similar properties was first realised at the Winter Olympic Games held in Nagano in 1998 where an enquiry was raised by a medical officer regarding whether the injection of insulin was strictly restricted to competing diabetic athletes (Sonksen, 2001). After realising insulin's anabolic, muscle building properties, its use in sport by non-diabetic individuals was swiftly banned by the International Olympic Committee in the same year. However, insulin has since been used widely among body builders, weigh lifters and power lifters to increase muscle mass and endurance (Rich et al, 1998; Tricker et al, 1989).

Despite the fact that insulin has been a prescription-only medicine since 1998, athletes can easily obtain the hormone through diabetic friends and relatives, and other unscrupulous online sources. Rich et al (1998) stated that athletes were regularly including insulin in their training regimes, injecting 10 units of long-acting insulin and eating high-carbohydrate foods to actively offset any hypoglycaemic effect on blood glucose levels. This practice is known as a hyperinsulinaemic clamp (Sonksen, 2001), where both glucose and insulin are present at the same time, effectively cancelling one-another out. The use of insulin in this way prevents any breakdown (catabolism) in muscle tissue and in the liver by increasing the production of glycogen and proteins, prompting the entry of glycogen and amino acids into the muscles before a competition (Evans and Lynch, 2003).

The use of insulin therefore allows a greater endurance in response to exercise because there is more glycogen available to fuel the muscles for longer. Unless the athlete is under medical supervision however, taking insulin when there is not a medical need, and taking any other anabolic substance to force new muscle growth, is a very dangerous practice. The extent to which some athletes are prepared to take risks with their health in order to win was shown in a survey in 1997 by Bamberger and Yaeger. The researchers asked elite athletes whether they would take performance-enhancing substances such as growth hormone, insulin-like growth factor-1 and insulin if they were guaranteed to definitely win over the other competitors, and they were guaranteed not to be caught. The results showed that 193 elite athletes would take the substance(s) and only three said that they would not take that risk. In a further question, the athletes were asked whether they would take a performance-enhancing substance if it guaranteed that they would win every competition they entered for the next five years, but then they would die from the side effects of taking the substance. The results showed that more than half of these elite athletes were prepared to take the risk of permanently damaging their bodies, resulting ultimately in death, in order to be seen as top in their chosen sporting discipline.

In addition to injecting several hormones known to increase muscle mass and strength, athletes also regularly took nutritional protein supplements for the same purpose of increasing the amount of protein available to be made into new muscle. Athletes have also stated that they perceived that taking nutritional supplements, in combination with strong anabolic androgenic steroids and growth hormone, helped them to recover from any type of muscle, ligament, tendon or even bone injury far more quickly. Sonksen (2001) has suggested that this may well be true and that this information is provided as fact in *The Underground Steroid Handbook* (Duchaine, 1983) which states that regular use of growth hormone strengthens tendons to the extent that damage from weight lifting and power lifting is significantly diminished. Sonksen (2001) has also stated that growth hormone may act to prevent stress fractures in this way, and also accelerates the healing process so that recovery from injury is far quicker, allowing the athlete to return to training and competition.

As mentioned earlier, growth hormone has the action of focussing nutritional calories into the production of protein and away from the production of fat. This has been seen in animal studies where increased growth hormone levels result in a greater percentage of lean body tissue and reduced fat stores. This is also the case in humans with the condition acromegaly (commonly known as giantism) where there is an over-production of growth hormone by the pituitary gland and excessive height as a result. In those with reduced levels of growth hormone, there is less lean body tissue and an increased fat mass (Sonksen, 2001). When recombinant (artificially manufactured) growth hormone is injected, there is a huge change in body composition, resulting in an average five kilogram increase in lean body mass in the first month in association with a five kilogram loss of fat mass, especially from around the abdominal organs (Salomon et al, 1989). These dramatic and quickly achieved physical changes make growth hormone use so popular and common in athletes, especially body builders, power lifters and weight lifters.

It has been known since 1916 that insulin has both a stimulating and inhibitory action in the body. Sir Edward Schafer (1916) proposed that insulin, which was not officially discovered until 1921 by Banting and Best, was a substance (he questioned the term "hormone") which had two important properties. Firstly, he described insulin as having certain "autoacid" actions (with stimulating properties) and secondly, he identified insulin as possessing inhibiting properties, or "chalones". He felt a lack of inhibitory actions (chalones) from insulin led to a failure to store glucose in the liver so the liver then overproduced glucose which accumulated in the blood, causing hyperglycaemia, specifically seen in cases of Type 1 diabetes (Sonksen, 2001). This, of course, could not be treated as there was no injectable insulin available at that time.

Later research in the 1950s demonstrated that insulin could stimulate the uptake of glucose into both the muscle and fat of rats, leading to the incorrect conclusion that high blood glucose levels in untreated diabetes are due to glucose not being able to enter the body cells to be used as fuel and, as a result, were pushed back into the blood. However, Sonksen (2001), an expert in the subject of insulin at Guy's, King's and St. Thomas' School of Medicine in London, states that glucose being able to enter muscle cells has now been shown not to be dependent on insulin. In actual fact, glucose can and does enter the body cells when there is hyperglycaemia, however, it cannot be metabolised as fuel when there is a lack of insulin.

As Schafer stated in 1916, insulin stimulates the transport of glucose from the cytoplasm (the jelly-like substance surrounding the nucleus of the cell) of muscle and fat tissue by increasing the amount of glucose transporters available. However, when there is an absence of insulin in the body there are still a number of glucose transporters present ensuring the cell has enough fuel to function (Sonksen, 2001). As mentioned earlier, insulin decreases glucose uptake in non-skeletal muscle. This is the case because the trigger for glucose uptake by muscle tissue is hyperglycaemia, as well as the concentration between intracellular and extracellular glucose levels (Sonksen and Sonksen, 2000). This is even the case in untreated Type 1 diabetes where there is no insulin being produced by the pancreas. In this state, glucose uptake in muscle tissue is increased by the lack of insulin, but not if severe diabetic ketoacidosis occurs (Sonksen, 2001), where protein begins to be burnt as fuel because the excess of glucose cannot then be utilised. However, what stops the cell's use of glucose during severe ketoacidosis is the products of the breakdown of protein (ketones) which prevent the metabolism of glucose, not the cell's inability to use glucose for fuel.

The regular use of insulin, obtained from sources such as those prescribed insulin to treat their Type 1 diabetes, has been admitted to be at least 10 percent of 450 body builders in a specific community (Evans and Lynch, 2003; Coglan, 2001). It is also an attractive substance because it disappears from the body very quickly and it can be difficult to distinguish from the athlete's own, naturally produced insulin. Insulin increases muscle bulk for athletes, body builders, power lifters and weight lifters in two ways. The presence of a raised amount of insulin in the blood stimulates amino acid transport in human skeletal muscle; it is also thought that this may have a role in muscle and amino acid protein metabolism (Banadonna et al, 1993).

As previously seen, insulin therefore promotes the entry of amino acids (the building blocks of proteins) into the body cells and enables the synthesis of proteins. Acting as a metabolic control, insulin regulates body systems such as anabolic effects and amino acid uptake. Amino acid uptake, which is controlled by insulin, also increases DNA replication. As mentioned earlier, insulin also decreases glucose uptake in non-skeletal muscle. Whilst insulin inhibits protein breakdown (the reason bodybuilders and power lifters take the hormone), bulk protein synthesis when there is injected insulin present only inhibits the breakdown of proteins when there is also an increase in amino acids (Banadonna et al, 1993). It has always been thought that the administration of insulin, without simultaneous food or glucose, lowers blood glucose levels because insulin reduces the amount of glucose taken up in the tissues such as muscle. Sonksen (2001) and Brown et al (1978) have stated that this is also a myth and that the action of insulin in diabetes, when there is no food or glucose present, actually inhibits the liver from producing glucose and does not stimulate peripheral uptake of glucose in the body.

### THE USE OF INSULIN BY SPORTS PERSONS IN PRACTICE

Whilst it has been well reported in the media that a wide proportion of amateur and elite individuals competitively participating in sport use performance-enhancing substances, there are fewer actual examples of the devastating and dangerous effects of this in practice (Evans and Lynch, 2003; Elkin et al, 1997; Tricker, 1989). Evans and Lynch (2003) have reported a case of a 31-year old male body builder who was found unconscious at his home and was them taken to the Accident and Emergency department of his local hospital. On examination he was found to be sweating profusely (a condition known as diaphoresis), but he was still breathing on his own, although this was very shallow, and the man was still withdrawing from pain when this reflex was tested. Despite this being an encouraging sign that his coma had not deepened to the stage where he did not respond to external stimuli, the man's eyes remained closed and he was at the level of unconsciousness where he did not speak. The man's rate of respiration was low, at only twenty breaths per minute, and his pulse was rapid, measured at a rate of 100 per minute. A blood glucose test measurement recorded as "low", meaning that this was too minimal to be recorded as a measurement by a standard blood glucose meter (usually this standard setting on the machine occurs with a level of <2mmol/L, or less than 36mg/dl). The unconscious man was immediately given a 50ml intravenous drip containing 50 percent dextrose (another name for glucose, termed D-glucose) and his hypoglycaemic condition rapidly improved.

Tests performed when the man arrived at the hospital showed that his low blood glucose had led to respiratory acidosis (a condition whereby decreased oxygen intake leads to a build up of carbon dioxide in the blood, reducing cell and tissue acidity to below 7.35 pH), with additional evidence of dehydration. Initial indications suggested that the patient may have Type 1 diabetes and be suffering from severe low blood glucose levels for this reason. However, once he was able to talk, the man confirmed that he was in fact a non-diabetic body builder who had been regularly taking long-acting insulin injections three times a week to increase his muscle bulk. The man had also been dieting strictly prior to a forthcoming completion and therefore had little or no stores of glycogen in his liver to offset his plummeting blood glucose levels due to these insulin injections.

Severe hypoglycaemia was caused by a combination of dieting and having recently changed the kind of insulin he was taking to a fast-acting type, presumably because he was obtaining the insulin from irregular sources such as someone with diabetes, and therefore he was unable to secure his usual long-acting variety. The fast-acting insulin taken with very little food was a disastrous combination. The body builder also stated that he took anabolic androgenic steroids to increase his muscle mass. This individual was lucky in that his lack of knowledge of the action of the different insulin working times did not lead to permanent damage, possibly because he was found by another person and quickly admitted to hospital to receive glucose before his brain struggled to maintain vital functions and was irreversibly affected. This highlights the issue that taking insulin when it is not medically recommended can lead to irreversible brain damage, sustained coma and potentially even death.

A second accidental insulin overdose which ended with far more serious consequences for the individual was reported by Elkin et al (1997). This was the case of a 21-year old male body builder who had been self-administering intravenous insulin in order to quickly build muscle mass, burn fat, and increase his muscle strength and endurance. In search of this desired result, this individual had turned to insulin use after taking anabolic steroids, a banned substance in sporting competition. He considered it to be too risky to continue with anabolic steroids in case he was caught and exposed as a cheat. The body builder discovered that insulin reportedly had similar anabolic effects on muscle to steroids without the additional worry of testing positively for a banned substance.

This risk-taking behaviour with little knowledge of the side effects of taking non-prescribed medicines recreationally, and in such a dangerous way, led to severe brain damage and lasting cognitive impairment as a result of prolonged hypoglycaemic coma because the individual took too much insulin. This case was reported by Elkin et al (1997) before the International Olympic Committee ban on non-diabetic athletes using insulin, although clearly this body builder thought insulin preferable and untraceable if he used it instead of anabolic steroids.

As seen previously, severe hypoglycaemia causes brain damage when there is a large dose of insulin working for several hours but no glucose to counteract its effects, where permanent damage to the brain results after the blood glucose level stays very low at 1.1mmol/L (20mg/dl) or less for five hours or more (Marks and Richmond, 2007). This is entirely possible if a body builder or weight lifter is training at home and they suddenly get into difficulty, collapsing and confused with severe hypoglycaemia, with no other persons present. Brain damage can be reversed if, following severe hypoglycaemic coma, blood glucose levels then remain within a normal range for several days, but lasting intellectual impairment results if hypoglycaemia is frequent.

Warren et al (2007) demonstrated that severe and recurrent hypogly-caemia leads to varying degrees of subsequent learning impairment, a reduction in the ability to understand and retain information, and lapses in memory concerning short-term events. Where severe hypoglycaemia has led to protracted coma, Magnetic Resonance Imaging scans have shown that there is permanent neurological dysfunction and structural abnormality of the brain, with the development of lesions in the frontal lobe and deep grey matter (Cranston, 2005). Other imaging studies have confirmed that when hypoglycaemia is severe, as in the case of the body builder reported by Elkin et al (1997), the brain goes into a state of shock with fitting occurring as a result. After the person recovers there is long-term cognitive (thought processes and patterns) impairment and lasting damage to the brain's cortex and hippocampus regions (Bree et al, 2009), whose normal function is to work quickly to retrieve memories. The case of the body builder highlighted by Elkin et al (1997) was unfortu-nate in that his self-administered intravenous insulin regime led to a severe depletion in blood glucose levels, leaving very lasting results. It is not known how many self-induced, milder hypoglycaemic incidents occur among athletes who abuse insulin, because without the need for hospitalisation they remain unreported, but this is potentially quite a prevalent occurrence.

Skårberg et al (2008) have provided a case report of six persons attending an addiction centre in Sweden after long-term use of anabolic androgenic substances, often accompanied by numerous other drugs to increase muscle mass in sport. Of these six individuals, two also included the use of insulin in their training regime for its anabolic effect. The first of these individuals began training at his local gym when he was 15 years of age and by the age of 16, he and his friends were only too aware of anabolic androgenic steroids and were keen to test their reputation. This adolescent was already taking dietary supplements such as protein compounds, creatine (a high-energy molecule found in the cells of skeletal muscle fibre) and multivitamins. This young amateur athlete then progressed to injecting testosterone into his buttocks which resulted in a marked increase in strength and body weight.

However, the young athlete also experienced the adverse effect of excess testosterone of increased irritability as he took more and more anabolic androgenic steroid products, also including testosterone derivatives by injection, and in tablet and fluid forms administered as drops under the tongue. Because anabolic androgenic steroids have the unwanted effect of producing breast tissue in males (a condition known as gynecomastia), this young man soon discovered that he could counteract this side-effect by also taking anti-oestrogen releasers, and that testosterone releasers would increase his natural testosterone production. In addition, this individual began to take growth hormone and insulin by injection in the hope of achieving even faster muscle growth. To this cocktail of drugs, he also added stimulants to perk him up, hormone boosters, and substances to prevent muscle breakdown.

As a result he was able to train for far longer and to push himself even harder, but this led to pronounced joint and muscle pain. Instead of seeing this as a sign that he should rest to prevent a serious sporting injury, the young man began to take regular doses of analgesic pain relief to mask his increasing discomfort. By the age of 20, this body builder was taking ten different human steroid substances in combination with testosterone releasers, insulin, and stimulants. Whilst he was happy with the muscle mass increase, ability and endurance effects he achieved, Skårberg et al (2008) have reported that this individual also experienced excessive hair growth on his back, skin lesions between his shoulders and on his chest musculature, acne, erectile dysfunction, wasting (atrophy) of the testicles, and a persistent cough that noticeably appeared worse after taking testosterone. As well as these unpleasant physical side-effects, he was affected by extreme jealousy, mood swings, poor memory, clinical depression and aggressiveness, and sadly also attempted suicide. Fortunately for this individual, his parents took action and contacted the addiction clinic because their son's physical appearance and personality had changed so dramatically.

The second case reported by Skårberg et al (2008) concerning insulin use in sport was that of another young male who developed an obsession with training at the gym at age 15. He became more and more interested in competing against other athletes to gauge his performance and, after several years, he began to express this competitive spirit in the discipline of body building. Because of the highly competitive aspect in this sport, this adolescent felt it necessary to take anabolic androgenic steroids in order to build muscle mass and increase his size and strength. This belief was driven by his perception that "everybody takes steroids in body building".

At the age of 20 he took his first oral anabolic steroids accompanied by injections of testosterone substances. This increased his muscle bulk and strength, making him feel "powerful". He also reported an increased sex drive and a feeling of self-confidence. Unfortunately this increased confidence and strength was not put to use in a good way, and the individual stated that he would deliberately pick fights to make himself feel good because of the power it gave him over others, making them afraid and scared of him. This unfortunate effect only served to feed his obsession to be bigger and stronger. Taking action, he researched the area of anabolic androgenic steroids further and discovered that testosterone releasers could be taken to enhance his natural testosterone production. In addition to anabolic steroids, this young man was also taking nutritional supplements such as protein compounds and creatine, the energy carrying molecule manufactured in all living cells.

The quest for even more substances to increase his muscle growth led this individual to inject himself with growth hormone, insulin and insulin-like growth factor-1. Over a total of four years he took a combination of nine different substances used in human and veterinary medicine. He also used stimulants to make him more alert, and took bronchodilators (taken by people with asthma to increase the size of their airway) in order to exploit their effect of reducing the amount of fat and fluid in the muscle tissue. The young body builder also dabbled with amphetamines (drugs which stimulate the central nervous system and induce a feeling of well-being and alertness, although they also increase the heart rate), along with recreational drugs such as hashish (dried hemp used for smoking or chewing), and occasional alcohol.

Due to the excessive use of insulin to build muscle mass, this individual experienced regular dramatic reductions in his blood glucose levels to the extent that he required hospitalisation on several occasions. This body builder fortunately recognised that his addiction and obsession with his body image had reached a serious stage where he needed professional help, so he decided to contact the addiction centre for treatment. Whilst undergoing this treatment however, he reportedly became fixated on the fact that he had lost four kilograms (just over eight and a half pounds) in weight, meaning he could not possibly return to his gym in future because he would be ridiculed by the other body builders. Unfortunately, he was also very depressed and felt it absolutely essential that he regained this lost weight quickly, so he began to take more anabolic steroids. This sadly resulted in numerous physical problems: breast development, acne, skin lesions, shrunken testicles, reduced sex drive and tiredness; and escalating psychological issues: worsening depression, mood swings, extreme aggression, frequent panic attacks, and an all-consuming obsession with his body image, leading him to finally decide to put a stop to his addictive behaviour.

Evans and Lynch (2003) have pointed out the dangers of body builders and power lifters taking insulin, especially when these individuals are not under medical supervision and are training alone. As previously seen by these examples, it is easy for excess insulin to act quickly without accompanying glucose or food prior to training. With a swift reduction in blood glucose levels cognitive function can reach a degree where the individual is no longer able to help themselves by eating or drinking something sweet to prevent the progression to severe hypoglycaemia and unconsciousness. In their papers, Coghlan (2001); Rich et al (1998); and Elkin et al (1997) have discussed the ease with which insulin can be obtained by non-diabetic sportspersons and used without medical supervision with dangerous consequences. Skårberg et al (2008) have raised awareness of how addictive patterns can easily develop in those who become obsessed with improving their personal and competitive performance at all costs.

It is clear that the use of performance-enhancing substances is driven by a desire to win, and keep on winning, no matter what. The use of these substances in sport must then be recognised as a psychological issue, similar to body dysmorphia (when the individual has an unrealistic, negative view of their body and how they appear to others). For the competing sports person wanting to be bigger, stronger and better than his or her peers, this obsessive drive encompasses many different factors such as body image, the perspective of how the athlete is viewed by peers, meeting personal motivations and goals, desire for success, the level of success achieved, and the search for continual improvement with the knowledge that certain substances can bring greater and faster results. These personal accounts of drug use in sport show that this can become a self-destructive, habit-forming, psychosocial process which may be incredibly difficult for the individual to move away from.

## THE CONSEQUENCES OF ENHANCING PERFORMANCE

As already seen in some of the case studies, long-term addiction and use of performance-enhancing drugs in sport can last for a number of years, requiring professional help to break the routine. Bamberger and Yaeger (1997) showed that the overwhelming drive to win at all costs was more important in the short-term for the vast majority of elite athletes, who may be paid large sums and be part of huge sponsorship deals, raising the pressure that they are under to perform. This has clear implications for taking these risks, despite the potential for the development of any long-term health problems due to the side effects of abusing drugs. The addictive and obsessive nature of competition means that more and more substance abuse is perceived to equal bigger and better results, so it is difficult to pinpoint any specific long term effects from taking one particular substance.

Insulin, as a medication for people with Type 1 diabetes, and those who take it because Type 2 diabetes medications no longer work effectively, do not suffer any particular adverse long-term changes in their overall health status as a consequence. It has been shown that individuals treated with insulin for diabetes have a lean body mass because of the effect of the hormone on muscle and fat composition when compared to people with diabetes who were not taking insulin as a medication (Singha et al, 1996). The acute short term side effect for people taking too much insulin, or insulin without food is, of course, hypoglycaemia. However, in most cases, this can be rapidly reversed with glucose and the brain and muscles recover remarkably quickly. With sustained severe hypoglycaemia however, sportsmen and women would experience eventual cognitive decline, such as memory loss and mental slowness.

Similarly, a study by Friedlander et al (2013) has shown that there are no long-term or adverse effects on the body in a study following a year of insulin-like growth factor-1 injections in post-menopausal women over age 60. Whilst this group is completely different from that of young, competing athletes, the researchers were looking at the effect of insulin-like growth factor-1 hormone replacement on body composition, bone density and psychological factors. Catabolism (chemical reactions that break down complex organic compounds into simple ones with the release of energy) slows down with age and this has been attributed to the ceasing of reproductive capability. The women were given regular injections of insulin-like growth factor-1 for one year at a level normally found in a healthy young person. The results showed that these booster injections did not alter body composition or blood levels of this hormone, bone density, strength, mood or memory to any significant degree. Therefore it is likely that similar results would be observed in athletes taking the same substance. However, insulin-like growth factor-1 is taken by athletes in combination with growth hormone in order to boost muscle bulk because the two hormones are believed to work in conjunction with one another.

Growth hormone does have a positive effect on fat and carbohydrate metabolism. However, Rennie (2003) has stated that there is no evidence of growth hormone promoting the retention of protein in muscle, but that this action is certainly possible in connective tissue. As a result, many body builders, weight lifters and athletes are putting themselves at risk of long-term chronic disease by injecting a substance with no positive benefit. Worryingly, the supposed effects of growth hormone are also being marketed as a rejuvenating substance for middle-aged and elderly men (Rennie, 2003), without openly stating the potential consequences of taking the hormone. Rennie (2003) has suggested that growth hormone is freely available to individuals online in the United States and that it can be bought in person in Mexico, having often been sourced on the black market, in some cases from cadavers, making it available to body building and professional athletic communities.

The promotion of the muscle building effects of growth hormone in the sporting media, and the continuing search by the International Olympic Committee for a means of definitively detecting such substances has elevated growth hormone to the status of being too good to be true if you want to be young, strong, and powerful. Whilst this hype has meant growth hormone is seen as a necessary boost to an athlete's training regime, in reality, regular use can lead to a poor athletic performance due to changes in the body's metabolism. As previously seen with the changes in hormone levels and their working times associated with poor sleep patterns, high levels of growth hormone taken in sport can also lead to heart irregularities, high blood pressure, insulin resistance and potentially Type 2 diabetes over time. Hormone levels in the body work in a fine balance together and if one substance is abnormally elevated or absent, this disrupts normal metabolic function, causing chronic health problems in the long-term.

The Danish Institute of Sports Medicine has studied endurance trained athletes who willingly took growth hormone (as opposed to be asked to take it for the purposes of research) in the belief that this would enhance their performance. The athletes found that there was a decrease in their exercise performance and that they were unable to complete cycling tasks that they were usually able to accomplish following the administration of growth hormone (Rennie, 2003). The Institute concluded that the reason for this was that growth hormone has the action of increasing lipolysis (the breakdown of lipids into fatty acids) occurring during exercise and that it also increased the amount of lactic acid produced by working muscles (Rennie, 2003). This reduced the rate of stored glucose available to the muscle tissue as fuel, making it more difficult to perform strenuous exercise and recover from it quickly.

As already seen, an excess of growth hormone, such as that used in the pursuit of sporting enhancement, is dangerous because it causes symptoms akin to the condition of acromegaly (giantism). Colago et al (2001) have shown that vastly increased amounts of growth hormone in

those with acromegaly led to poor exercise tolerance, which improved
after treatment to reduce levels of this hormone produced by the pituitary
gland. Khaleeli et al (1984) have shown that individuals suffering from
acromegaly do not have an increased muscle size in relation to their
greater height, but do experience multiple changes in muscle fibre
composition, including atrophy (wasting). In addition, acromegaly is
commonly accompanied by cardiovascular disease, Type 2 diabetes,
irregular fat metabolism, osteoarthritis, and breast and colon cancers
(Rennie, 2003; Jenkins, 2001). For those with this condition there is also a
greater possibility of sudden death due to irregular heart rhythm (cardiac
arrhythmia), and an increased chance of contracting Creutzfeldt-Jakob
disease (Rennie, 2003) from growth hormone extracted from cadavers,
a condition also known as spongiform encephalopathy, causing rapid
deterioration of the brain and progressive dementia.

There are several health conditions where the administration of growth
hormone can be of benefit. These include children with growth defects
(Fine et al, 2000; Germak, 1996); children suffering from kidney failure
(Haffner et al, 2001); and babies who are born underweight for their
gestational age (Leger et al, 1998). Studies of older people who are deficient
in growth hormone and are treated with this hormone also have positive
effects, with an increased rate of muscle protein use (Butterfield et al,
1997), and a reduction in body fat, encouraging lean body mass (Cuneo
et al, 1991; Cuneo et al, 1992; Salomen et al, 1989). As the name suggests,
growth hormone is of benefit for people who are deficient in this area
due to medical conditions. Growth hormone taken by young, fully grown
individuals as an aid to increasing muscle mass and strength does not
produce the same positive effects.

Many animal studies have demonstrated that growth hormone does
increase muscle mass and boosts muscle size and strength when training
and exercising. However, Rennie (2003) has pointed out that these studies
were not carried out on human subjects (as this would be unethical)
and that the animals involved were probably still growing, hence the

increase in size and sensitivity to the effects of growth hormone. It has been reported that human growth hormone administration increases the amount of amino acids (the building blocks of protein) present in the forearms of athletes due to the stimulation of protein use by the body, but not by preventing protein from being broken down (Fryberg et al, 1995; Fryberg et al, 1991). There is little long-term change in protein synthesis as a result of injecting growth hormone in healthy subjects and once injections cease, this effect no longer occurs. Rennie (2003) has emphasised that there are no credible studies of muscle protein use, body composition change or increased strength in young to middle-aged, healthy subjects to support the injection of growth hormone by athletes to enhance their performance.

If it is the case that growth hormone injections have no effect on muscle mass in athletes hoping to exploit the belief that the opposite is true, there must be some measurable effect in order to continue taking it. Rennie (2003) has suggested that athletes take growth hormone for several reasons. As growth hormone has the effect of changing the balance of water and salt in the muscles and joints, there is a palpable difference for athletes after injecting the hormone. Rennie (2003) has stated that this change is perceived as a positive increase in muscle mass, therefore reinforcing the idea that growth hormone should continue to be taken to achieve this effect. Growth hormone also has the action, as previously seen, of channelling calories consumed in food into the production of protein rather than fat, therefore creating a leaner body mass if taken regularly. This fast reduction in subcutaneous (under the skin) fat deposits is perceived by athletes as due to muscle enhancement as muscle definition becomes more apparent Rennie (2003).

However, this definition is not due to any increase in muscle size. It is also unlikely that an elite athlete would have a high body fat mass as they tend to be lean, with the exception of some weight and power lifters. This change in fat to muscle ratio achieved with the injection of growth hormone does not actually enhance sporting performance.

Rennie (2003) has suggested that the effect of persuasive hype about the positive properties of growth hormone on young athletes who want quick results is to blame for the hormone's miraculous reputation. This is fuelled by the fact that growth hormone is now a banned substance, decided by the International Olympic Committee, despite it having no measurable positive effect on sporting performance in healthy young persons. This makes the emphasis on developing a test which will detect the use of growth hormone by athletes nonsensical as there is little point in doing so, given that the hormone does not enhance performance. In addition, growth hormone does not stay in the athlete's system for long enough to reach the urine, so it has to be tested for in blood.

The substances that are well reported to produce a muscle mass enhancement effect are anabolic androgenic steroids. As seen in the previous case studies of young athletes taking multiple steroid substances, this resulted in the development of increased aggression and severe psychological problems. This is because anabolic androgenic steroids are produced from derivatives of testosterone, the male hormone produced in the testes from puberty (Tortora and Grabowski, 1993). Testosterone is both anabolic, in that it builds new muscle, and has androgenic properties, meaning that it is responsible for the development of masculine characteristics.

As well as its role in puberty, testosterone has many functions in the body, including regulating the metabolism of protein in muscles, sexual and cognitive functions, the formation of red blood cells, and the metabolism of fats in plasma and bone (Evans, 2004). Whilst steroids have both anabolic and androgenic effects on the body, purified anabolic steroids have attempted to separate the two actions for use in sport, concentrating on the anabolic action. Non-purified, anabolic androgenic steroids have some positive medical effects in certain cancers such as leukaemia, HIV, under-developed gonads in adult males, and kidney and liver failure (Basaria et al, 2001). However, as seen earlier with growth hormone abuse in sport, taking testosterone derivatives has detrimental effects such as skin lesions, excess hair growth, acne, aggression, depression, and mood swings.

In the UK, anabolic androgenic steroids are classed as a prescription-only drug under the Medications Act, 1968; they are also class C controlled drugs under the Misuse of Drugs Act, 1971. In the USA, the Anabolic Steroid Control Act was introduced in 2004 due to the increased abuse of these substances by athletes. Because of the known dramatic side effects of anabolic androgenic steroid use, many athletes have tailored their dosages using three common methods to avoid adverse consequences: "cycling", "stacking", and "pyramiding" (Lukas, 2003). "Cycling" involves an athlete taking steroid for a number of weeks, then stopping them for a set time before recommencing them once more. "Stacking" involves the individual using several steroid substances simultaneously but varying the administration method, such as injection, then tablet form in the hope of fooling the body into not reacting adversely to the dosages. "Pyramiding" is the process of repeatedly building up to a maximum dosage of steroids, then reducing the dose back down again in order for the body to adjust to the differing hormonal levels. Whilst these methods have varying success in avoiding side-effects, some athletes chose to take even more drugs to counteract these known side- effects, such as medications to prevent breast development.

There are a number of significant psychological side-effects associated with taking anabolic androgenic steroids, but there are few scientific studies exploring these multiple problems as a whole and therefore, there is no consistently proven link. Physical aggression has been shown to increase dramatically when testosterone-based steroids are taken, and this has been observed in research studies and, as seen earlier, this has also been self-reported by athletes (Eisenberg and Galloway, 2005; Copeland et al, 2000). An increase in aggressive behaviour occurs with moderately small doses of testosterone, as does an increase in irritability, mood swings, hostility and violence towards others (Su et al, 1993). Lukas (2003) has also reported several accounts of "roid rage" where individuals have exhibited frenzied, violent behaviour whilst taking high doses of anabolic steroids.

Another study by Dukarm et al (1996) has examined the behaviour of teenagers taking testosterone-based anabolic steroids and has reported triple the incidence of serious violent episodes as a result. There has also been a high incidence of psychotic symptoms (grandiose and paranoid states) reported by those taking steroids (Pope and Katz, 1994; 1988). Other consequences of taking anabolic androgenic steroids (derivatives of testosterone) concern their long-term effects of these on muscles, tendons and bone. Increased muscle mass has been associated with over-stressing of the tendons and muscles so that they become injured more easily; testosterone also has the effect of prematurely fusing the growth plates (epiphyses) in the long bones of adolescents, leading to a shorter stature (Liow and Tavares, 1995).

Damage to the heart, such as enlargement of the left ventricle, and cardiac

arrhythmia (altered heart rhythm) has also been widely reported in association with steroid use, as has high blood pressure, and increased blood clotting (Urhausen et al, 2004; Kutscher et al, 2002). Urhausen et al (2004) have demonstrated that, even after stopping anabolic steroid use for a number of years, the left ventricle remained enlarged in the body builders and powers lifters studied. Eisenberg and Galloway (2005) also reported adverse effects in the liver, leading to jaundice and tumours in some individuals who had taken anabolic androgenic steroids.

With relevance to the additional injection of insulin are the effects that anabolic steroids have on the endocrine system. Insulin resistance (losing sensitivity to insulin so that more needs to be produced by the pancreas) has been reported in women taking testosterone-based steroids (Diamond et al, 1998) which can lead to Type 2 diabetes long-term, but a further study has conversely shown that this is not always the case in men (Hobbs et al, 1996). Women who take anabolic androgenic steroids have experienced masculinisation of their features, breast shrinkage, unwanted hair growth, and a deepening of their voice (Rashid et al, 2007). Because injection is the primary method of administering anabolic steroids, growth hormone, testosterone, insulin and insulin-like growth factor-1, users sharing needles risk contracting the HIV virus, hepatitis B and C. However, a study by Crampin et al (1998) showed that only two percent of 149 individuals studied who injected steroids over a five-year period were hepatitis B positive, compared with 18 percent of heroin users, suggesting athletes were aware of keeping their injection equipment sterile.

## CATCHING THE CHEATERS

In 2002, the Bay Area Laboratories Co-Operative (BALCO) scandal was uncovered. This began in a vitamin shop in Milbrae, California, which would diagnose and treat mineral deficiencies in athletes, and carry out blood and urine analysis. It escalated to a major provider of performance-enhancing substances. From 1996 the owner, Victor Conte, with the aid of an enterprising chemist and a distributor, successfully provided nutritional supplements to get athletes to the peak of fitness and his client list grew to include professional sportspersons. Conte marketed this special concoction of various "undetectable" drugs which were then manufactured and distributed illegally.

These substances included insulin; growth hormone; testosterone cream (designed specifically for the purpose of introducing testosterone to the body); erythropoietin (responsible for the production of red blood cells); Modafinil, to be taken before competition, (prescribed medically as a mild stimulant for the condition of narcolepsy, where individuals continually and spontaneously fall asleep for very short periods throughout the day); tetrahydrogestrinone (a designer anabolic steroid substance); and other substances (Fainaru-Wada and Williams, 2006). Conte and his unscrupulous chemist refined the use of these substances to the extent that, when used in rotation, they were virtually undetectable when tested. This method is similar to the "cycling" technique used by athletes to prevent the side-effects of anabolic androgenic steroids, involving an athlete taking a steroid(s) for a period of six to twelve weeks, then stopping administration for a set time before recommencing them once more.

The assurance by Conte that his combined substance was undetectable became, naturally, very attractive to many amateur and elite athletes. In 2002 an official federal investigation began into this co-operative, and in 2003, the United States Drug Agency received a syringe containing a small sample of this substance, reportedly gained from a locker-room floor (Mukhapadyay, 2007) from a sprint coach, allowing a separate investigation to be mounted. This was tested by Don Catlin, founder of the UCLA Olympic Analytical Laboratory, who had previously developed a test for tetrahydrogestrinone, one of the substances included in Conte's concoction. Don Catlin tested 550 existing samples from athletes and discovered that 20 of these were positive for the steroid.

A number of athletes were then discredited for using this substance, including British 100 metre sprinter, Dwaine Chambers, who was barred for life from competing in the Olympics and was given a two-year ban from entering any competition. Legal action was taken. The BALCO scandal was widely reported and had lasting repercussions in all sports, particularly baseball, where new policies were introduced. Victor Conte now runs a company called Scientific Nutrition for Advanced Conditioning after receiving and serving a four-month prison sentence in 2005 (Fainaru-Wada and Williams, 2006). He no longer sells illegal substances. Conte's co-conspirators, the chemist and distributor, each received a three-month prison sentence for their involvement.

The BALCO case illustrates how anabolic androgenic substances may be tailored to slip under the testing radar, and the levels to which athletes will go because they want to win without detection. As a result, designated persons are now assigned the task of collecting blood and urine samples from athletes for testing in the event that a sample is swapped or tampered with. There have been examples of a urine sample being switched for a drug-free one; the use of watered-down urine, forcing sporting facilities to have to switch water off at the mains when testing occurs; and even the use of a prosthetic device to hold artificial urine (Mukhapadyay, 2007). These samples are taken regularly from athletes and they are strictly guarded when they are taken to the laboratory for testing, and once they arrive (Mukhapadyay, 2007). The samples are labelled, but not with the athlete's name (as this is not provided) in case this may influence the person testing the urine and blood provided. There are hundreds of banned substances which may be tested for, including anabolic steroids, stimulants, hormones, and even whole blood transfusions (Mukhapadyay, 2007). The scientists testing the samples do not test for any specific substance unless they are asked to do so, beginning by testing the acidity and density. Large compounds are then identified, for example, anabolic steroids. This means that testing facilities have banks of reference materials to set a baseline regarding how a substance will appear in the laboratory. Laboratories also readily share knowledge and databases when new substances are introduced by athletes who hope to cheat this stringent system.

In an effort to cheat the testing process, some athletes have attempted to obscure a positive test result. Athletes may ingest various other substances with their performance-enhancing drugs which have the same spectroscopy retention times in order to deliberately interfere with the analysis (Mukhapadyay, 2007). Another method of cheating the testing process is to take diuretic substances so that the urine sample provided is watered down, in the hope that any trace of the banned substance will be undetected, or to tamper with a urine sample using substances (proteases) to breakdown proteins from hormone misuse (Mukhapadyay, 2007). Two samples from each athlete are provided and, if one proves positive without question, the laboratory reports this to the relevant anti-doping organisation responsible for the competitors. This organisation will then identify the athlete who provided the sample which has been found positive for a banned substance. Because athletes do not openly admit to cheating, the second sample is then tested for the same substance. This second test is witnessed by the athlete in question and their legal representative. If the second sample is also found to contain the banned substance, the athlete is presumed to be guilty of cheating and the appropriate action is taken.

As previously seen, Rennie (2003) has stated that the development of a reliable test to detect growth hormone is completely unnecessary as growth hormone has no effect on muscle mass and strength in healthy, fully grown adults. The development of a test to detect the misuse of insulin however has become necessary due to the substantial increase in athletes injecting insulin to enhance performance, confident that this will not be detected. Another problem facing doping control bodies was the difficulty in identifying any difference between synthetically-produced insulin and endogenous insulin (produced by the athlete's own pancreas). Traditionally, the detection of insulin in blood samples has been achieved using techniques which can trace a very small amount of insulin in a blood sample. Nuclear physicists, Rosalyn Yalow and Solomon Berson were awarded a Nobel Prize for Medicine in 1960 for developing this technique using radioactive insulin and antibody studies (called radioimmunoassay), which was able to measure tiny amounts of insulin (reacting only with the antibody) in blood and tissues. This technique was later found to be often unreliable, being subject to reaction with other molecules, and sometimes creating artefacts (Marks and Richmond, 2007), making some results questionable. This meant that laboratory testing procedures needed to emphasise the importance of recognising what information was being given by a specific antibody; and that a policy must be in place if two separate antibodies were identified in two different tests to ensure that any reaction with other molecules did not lead to false results. Certain hormones are still tested for using immunoassay antibody detection techniques. In addition to insulin, human chorionic gonadotropin and luteinising hormone, controlling growth and reproduction, are taken by athletes because they have the effect of increasing testosterone production. Human chorionic gonadotropin is also secreted by some tumours (Mukhapadyay, 2007), and these have been detected in athletes undergoing immunoassay testing for substance misuse.

In the 2004 Olympic Games in Athens, a greater number of athletes were found to have been taking performance-enhancing substances than ever before. This is because new and more sensitive testing methods were introduced which discovered the cheating. Athletes may have used the substances in order to boost their performance so they were chosen for their Olympic team, staying clear of taking the substances for several days before testing was undertaken. More recently, mass spectrometry testing has been introduced in order to detect long-acting insulin usage by non-diabetic athletes in urine samples. It was once the case that naturally-produced and synthetically designed hormones, such as testosterone, could not be distinguished using mass spectroscopy techniques (Mukhapadyay, 2007). However, a method was developed which identified the constituent compound of synthetic testosterone to originate from plants (typically yams), which was then converted into testosterone; human testosterone having a different carbon isotope (Mukhapadyay, 2007).

Thomas et al (2007) developed a mass spectrometry test to identify the products of the degradation (breakdown) of the long-acting insulins known as Lantus, Insulin Glargine, Levemir, and Insulin Detemir. The researchers found definitive products of the breakdown of Lantus insulin in the urine samples provided. However, the procedure was not able to clearly identify degradation products for Insulin Glargine, Levemir or Insulin Detemir. Whilst this is disappointing, this research does bring the identification of insulin breakdown products closer. The researchers have stated that, because synthetic insulins are modified, there are a number of different amino acid degradation products and these, once recognised, can be identified with mass spectrometry. Athletes who inject long-acting insulin for its anabolic properties may therefore now choose to take either Glargine, Levemir or Insulin Detemir, which are currently difficult to detect using mass spectrometry techniques

The use of performance-enhancing substances in sport will always continue, as it has done since the first Olympic Games in ancient Greece, while athletes seek ways in which they can be better than the competition. Mukhapadyay (2007) has suggested that drug users in sport may be caught more widely than by simply testing them for banned substances prior to competition by using methods such as collaborating with law-enforcement agencies who have information about drug dealers and their contacts. Whistle-blowing by honest athletes also helps keep sport clean as the cheaters are publically identified by their peers and banned from the sport of their choice, potentially altering their whole life as a consequence, as in the case of Lance Armstrong.

Health education is very important in sport, especially for younger athletes, with an emphasis on the serious side-effects of drug taking. It has been shown that growth hormone has no positive effect in the healthy, fully-grown body on muscle strength and mass, but the myth that it can enhance performance, and the emphasis on developing a test to catch those taking it, perpetuates its use. It is also the case that a competition won purely because of cheating rather than by effort is a hollow victory and, even if the athlete gets away with it, he or she knows that it is not an achievement based on their personal ability.

CHAPTER FOUR

# ABUSING INSULIN
# TO LOSE WEIGHT

The abuse of insulin is not only confined to the exploitation of its anabolic properties in sport. Those who have been prescribed insulin for the purpose of treating their Type 1 diabetes may also misuse it in order to achieve rapid weight loss. This practice is known as diabulimia, but this is not a diagnosis accepted by many health professionals. Diabulimia is not a condition recognised by the medical profession, although it is believed to affect one-third of women with Type 1 diabetes (Wilson, 2012). It is periodically reported in the media (Elkins, 2012; Wark, 2007) and in academic circles (Shaban, 2013; Young et al, 2013; Goebel-Fabbri et al, 2008; Colton et al, 2007), among others).

Diabulimia is a practice which involves the individual choosing to deliberately under-dose or completely omit their insulin treatment in order to induce a state of ketoacidosis due to high blood glucose levels (hyperglycaemia).This altered and dangerous metabolic state induces rapid weight loss and, for this reason, this deliberate diabetes mis-management is considered to be an eating disorder (Ruth-Sahd et al, 2010; 2009). Many, but not most, women with Type 1 diabetes realise that they have a unique way of drastically manipulating their weight by restricting their insulin dosages, and Ruth-Sahd et al (2010; 2009) have stated that a proportion of women have deliberately done this at some point in their lives.

Insulin deficiency can be due to the development of Type 1 diabetes, as a result of the lack of administration of insulin (absolute deficiency), or as a consequence of under-dosing and failure to meet metabolic need (relative deficiency). The body cannot metabolise glucose effectively without insulin. Diabetic ketoacidosis results when there is a complete lack of or insufficient insulin present, with an associated increase in counter-regulatory hormones such as glucagon, cortisol and epinephrine. Hormonal imbalance triggered by the lack of insulin increases the presence of triglycerides (fats) and the catabolism of muscle, metabolised as an alternative source of fuel.

As the body is effectively not getting enough glucose as a primary source of fuel for its cells, the liver begins the process of trying to correct this deficiency. Glycerol and alanine (non-carbohydrate carbon substrates) are generated by the liver in the process known as hepatic gluconeogenesis to produce glucose; and glycogenolysis (the breakdown of glycogen by the liver to release stored glucose), leading to severe hyperglycaemia (Savage et al, 2011). Increased lipolysis (the breakdown of lipids) and glucagon in the lack of insulin raise serum free fatty acids resulting in the production of a large amount of ketone bodies by the liver, creating a state of metabolic acidosis.

Hyperglycaemia induces osmotic diuresis (urine production) leading to marked loss of water and electrolytes in the urine, and the accompanying ketosis leads to nausea and vomiting resulting in fluid depletion, severe dehydration and electrolyte imbalance. The condition of diabetic ketoacidosis results in a significant number of deaths; mortality being between one and 10 percent (Wright et al, 2009) and more than 20 percent of people with Type 1 diabetes experience frequent episodes of hyperglycaemia and ketoacidosis (Joint British Diabetes Society Guidelines for the Management of Diabetic Ketoacidosis, 2010). Attributing these cases to a cause such as deliberate under-dosing of insulin in diabulimia is, of course, very difficult.

Because an increased number of ketone bodies are produced when glucose cannot be used as a source of energy, a large amount of body weight can be lost in a very short time. This process can occur during illness and not as a deliberate weight loss strategy, when the need for insulin may increase three-fold (Jarvis and Rubin, 2003) but a correct dosage is not given because the individual is unaware that they have this increased need. Women wishing to lose weight may, however, seize upon this "miracle" technique and use it to periodically shed weight quickly thereafter. Shaw and Favazza (2010) suggest that the condition, or diabulimic behaviour, is present in 14 percent of adolescents with Type 1 diabetes, whilst Kelly et al (2005) have estimated that this figure is 16 percent at any one time, and have stated that as many as half of women with diabetes also had some type of eating disorder.

Alternative studies including diabulimia with other eating disorder behaviour have stated a figure of 27 percent (Young et al, 2013; Smith et al, 2008; National Institute for Care Excellence [NICE], 2004); and 36 percent (Peveler et al, 2005) prevalence respectively. It is thought that adolescent females diagnosed with Type 1 diabetes are at a greater risk of developing eating disorders than non-diabetic females in this age group because they are very conscious of their body image and gain weight once their diabetes is stabilised with insulin treatment, making them vulnerable (Ackard et al, 2008).

Insulin dosages may be forgotten rather than deliberately omitted if the individual has not developed a regular routine to manage their recently-diagnosed condition. It must also be remembered that blood glucose levels may be very erratic because of particularly difficult to control Type 1 diabetes, especially relevant in adolescence where insulin requirements are increased and insulin sensitivity is reduced during puberty (Amiel et al, 1986). With these various factors making Type 1 diabetes hard to control, resulting in hyperglycaemia and potentially leading to ketoacidosis, recognition of diabulimia as a choice by the individual may be difficult to identify.

The Diabetes Control and Complications Trial (1993; 1995) identified a causal link between consistently high levels of blood glucose and the development of chronic complications such as eye disease (retinopathy); kidney disease (nephropathy); nerve damage (neuropathy); heart and artery disease (macrovascular disease); and damage to the small blood vessels (microvascular disease). The psychological disorder of diabulimia is a deliberate mis-management of a serious chronic health condition which has the above long-term consequences. By inducing diabetic ketoacidosis with a state of continual hyperglycaemia, the body is flung into a state of shock where the metabolism of glucose is impaired and the cells must seek an alterative source of fuel.

Repeated episodes of diabetic ketoacidosis and poor metabolic control have been shown to be definitively associated with the onset of diabetic retinopathy (Mohamed et al, 2007; Rydall et al, 1997), the delicate blood vessels at the back of the eyes being one of the first areas of the body to be affected by ongoing hyperglycaemia. Retinopathyis a chronic complication of diabetes which describes a number of symptoms including abnormal dilation of the blood vessels of the eyes and haemorrhages of the retina. In advanced cases the retina becomes heavily scarred and this may lead to blindness (Shotliff and Duncan, 2005; Colas et al, 1991). Nephropathy (damage to the nephrons of the kidneys), is often seen in conjunction with the development of retinopathy. Nephropathy is a chronic complication of diabetes caused by persistently high blood glucose levels leading to hardening of the kidney tissue and changes in the structure of the tubular epithelial cells of the kidneys (MacIsaac and Watts, 2005).

Deliberate under-dosing of prescribed insulin to maintain a state of hyperglycaemia therefore brings both short and long-term acute and chronic health problems and a major deterioration in quality of life.

The individual's overall desire and unique ability to manipulate their body weight through insulin misuse is a complex (both metabolically and psychologically) and very dangerous practice. People have died by deliberately omitting their insulin for this purpose (Elkins, 2012; Goebel-Fabbri et al, 2008), and others have triggered devastating complications which they are then forced to live with (Wilson, 2012).

## A UNIQUE EATING DISORDER

Three main eating disorder patterns have been classified according to the DSM IV-TR criteria of eating disorders (Cleveland Clinic, 2011): anorexia, where there is an obsessive fear of gaining weight resulting in severe dietary restriction; bulimia, a disorder characterised by binge eating, then vomiting or laxative abuse; and unspecified eating disorders exhibiting some of these symptoms. Manipulating insulin dosages in order to lose weight actually falls under the category of bulimia nervosa (an overwhelming desire to eat a lot of food, followed by induced vomiting and taking quantities of laxatives to avoid weight gain). Diabulimia is a difficult and upsetting condition, and is also referred to in the literature as disordered eating rather than as an eating disorder in its own right in the context of adolescent females with Type 1 diabetes. Eating disorders occur less frequently in young males than they do in young females, measured at 1 in every 400 males, compared with 1 in 50 females (NICE, 2004). Diabulimia is seen even less often in diabetic males.

Because there is no diabetes-specific measure of the condition, it is difficult to assess the prevalence of diabulimia, but available figures suggest that this might be as high as 27 percent in terms of meeting the criteria for bulimia nervosa, including binge eating disorder (Young et al, 2013; Smith et al, 2008; NICE, 2004); whilst Peveler et al (2005) found that the figure was 36 percent. In addition to the dangers of inducing diabetic ketoacidosis in order to lose weight, this behaviour has also been found to be accompanied by binge eating, bulimia (inducing vomiting and misuse of laxatives) and excessive exercise (which can induce hyperglycaemia when there is insufficient insulin) by more young females suffering with Type 1 diabetes (eight percent) when compared with one percent of non-diabetic girls (Smith et al, 2008; Colton et al, 2004).

Other studies have concentrated on the long-term consequences of diabulimia at eight and 12-year follow-up intervals (Goebel-Fabbri et al, 2008; Colton et al, 2007; Colton et al, 2004). Inevitably, by restricting insulin and inducing hyperglycaemia over a number of years, these young women had developed peripheral neuropathy (nerve damage), a complex condition affecting the feet and hands. Peripheral neuropathy is a chronic complication of diabetes which occurs in two types: diffuse neuropathy, commonly appearing as disorders of sensation in the extremities of the body, and distal polyneuropathy, affecting many nerves of the hands and feet. The study also found that restricting insulin to lose weight increased the incidence (the rate of increase) of death by 3.2 times (Goebel-Fabbri et al, 2008). The desire to reduce insulin dosages may also be connected with the fear of severe hypoglycaemia which, as previously mentioned, can be very frightening, where the individual feels that they are unable to control what is happening to them as they must rely on another person when glucose levels are so low that the individual cannot help themselves.

Although it is not known why an individual diagnosed with the serious condition of Type 1 diabetes may choose to induce life-threatening complications by restricting their insulin dosages, there are some common factors which make this more likely. As already seen, diabulimia is far more common in female adolescents wishing to control their weight. This has also been linked to the necessary dietary restraints imposed by a diagnosis of Type 1 diabetes: having to monitor the carbohydrate content of food and calculate the correct insulin dosage in order to maintain normal blood glucose levels. Other factors which make diabu-limic behaviour more likely are weight gain following commencement of insulin treatment for Type 1 diabetes [reversing hyperglycaemia and due to the anabolic action of insulin, and because insulin induces hunger]; low self-esteem [which accompanies the diagnosis of a chronic disease, marking the adolescent as different from their peers]; and if there is dysfunction within the family setting [which may occur due to the high demands of accommodating a diagnosis of Type 1 diabetes into the usual routine and lifestyle] (Shaban, 2013).

Because Type 1 diabetes involves the sufferer being highly vigilant about the food they eat (including the ingredients that go into bought food), the portion sizes, and the restrictive element of what should and should not be eaten, diabulimia is in effect a control issue (of body weight and of the condition that imposes these rules), albeit having negative consequences. For this reason, diabulimia is not usually confined to one or two incidences of deliberately restricting insulin dosage; longitudinal studies showing that this behaviour can last for many years (Goebel-Fabbri, 2008; Colton et al, 2007; Colton et al, 2004). A study carried out by Neumark-Sztainer (2002) discovered that among women and men with Type 1 diabetes, regular under-dosing with insulin was the most favoured method of weight control.

Not surprisingly, a study which asked adolescent females with Type 1 diabetes if they had ever been overweight found that this factor was the most likely reason to engage in diabulimic behaviour (Markowitz et al, 2010). It is more likely for adolescent females with Type 1 diabetes to have a higher body mass index than those without diabetes (Starkey and Wade, 2010; Domargard et al, 1999) because insulin lays down fat stores and, as previously seen, induces hunger; plus the insulin dosage must be "fed" with a certain amount of carbohydrates to avoid low blood glucose levels, especially when exercising. A history of weight problems has therefore been highlighted as a strong indicator for omitting insulin to achieve weight control (Olmstead et al, 2008).

This may also be reinforced by the emphasis on weight as a person with Type 1 diabetes, and regularly being weighed by the GP, Practice Nurse and at the diabetes clinic, which can mean this issue becomes over-emphasised by health professionals and can lead to adverse reactions if weight gain or excess weight is perceived as a criticism. This is especially relevant for adolescent females, with low self-esteem and a high awareness of their body image and how others see them. Grylli et al (2005) found that when comparing adolescent females without eating disorders with other young women with Type 1 diabetes who had disordered eating behaviour, the latter had fewer positive attitudes, they perceived that they had more problems, had a lower level of self-esteem, and showed a higher rate of depression.

Certain indicators of diabulimic behaviour, and poor diabetes self-management among adolescent females have been recognised, including the absence of finger-prick marks indicating a lack of regular home blood glucose testing and diabetes self-management behaviour; infrequent orders for insulin on prescription; weight loss, or fluctuating body weight; erratic HbA1c measurements [venous blood tests which show the amount of glucose sticking to the red blood cells over a three-month period]; changes in mood and depressive behaviour (Ruth-Sahd et al, 2009). Recognition of these changes requires someone to know the individual well enough to notice, which is often not the case with health professionals who are not visited on a regular basis, and if there is a high staff turnover.

Research has suggested that having a chronic medical condition is a factor that makes associated eating disorders more likely. This area is clearly contentious, as living with one chronic disease is not the same as living with another, making this difficult to compare. Variables such as the individual's own coping strategies, the level of pain experienced, the individual's health beliefs, acceptance of the condition and its confines, depression, motivation and the amount of self-care required to manage the disorder all impact on outcome. However, Smith et al (2008) attempted such a comparison of adolescent females with scoliosis (curvature of the spine) and those with Type 1 diabetes in relation to rates of disordered eating, comparing the eating behaviour of those with a chronic disease to the eating behaviour seen among healthy adolescent young women. The study showed, unsurprisingly, that the adolescents with Type 1 diabetes were more likely to have an eating disorder than those with scoliosis or with no health problems at all, although all participants were categorised as being overweight or obese.

As Type 1 diabetes imposes strict dietary requirements on the individual from the age of diagnosis, which has a peak incidence of developing at age 10–14 years, Type 1 diabetes is a condition clearly linked to diet, control, restriction, and vigilance regarding choice and amount of food, (for example, going out with friends as an adolescent female with Type 1 diabetes and eating a high carbohydrate meal, requiring a large dose of insulin, because the individual does not want to be the odd one out). The author, having Type 1 diabetes from the age of 10, distinctly recalls being strictly lectured by health professionals about what was permissible to eat, and what was not, and in what restricted quantity. The graphically explained consequences of dying of kidney failure, going blind, or having my legs amputated if I did not comply stay with me to this day. Whilst diabetes health education has fortunately moved on from this scare tactics technique, the emphasis on food is always present for those with diabetes (both Type 1 and Type 2), which is not the case in the condition of scoliosis, other than that obesity does not help spinal curvature. Therefore, Type 1 diabetes is unique in the high self-care demands it imposes on the individual and the toll it takes on health in the short and long-term.

## DIABULIMIA IN PRACTICE

As a female with Type 1 diabetes from childhood, and now as a diabetes health educator, the subject of diabulimia interests me greatly. I have spoken at length with many other women like myself over the years, and found that the vast majority had quickly discovered the ease with which rapid weight loss could be achieved during a state of ketoacidosis. In most cases this was at first not deliberate: high blood glucose levels had occurred as a result of infection and the lack of emphasis, in the 1970s, that much more insulin, possibly three times normal dosage (Jarvis and

Rubin, 2003) is required during infection when blood glucose levels can become hugely increased.

Hyperglycaemia in association with infection is thought to be due to the invading bacteria adversely affecting glucose metabolism. Although the relationship between hyperglycaemia and the development of chronic complications of diabetes was not definitively confirmed until the Diabetes Control and Complications Trial (1993; 1995), specific tissue damage caused by high blood glucose levels was actually first recognised as the ultimate cause of chronic complications as early as 1930. As a result of this perceived lack of knowledge, one woman told the author that her doctor (GP rather than diabetes consultant) had actually suggested that she took less insulin when she was a teenager in the mid-1980s as this would help her to lose weight. When this woman questioned this many years later with a diabetes nurse (having later developed diabetic eye disease and peripheral nerve damage), the nurse replied that health professionals simply had not known how damaging high blood glucose levels were at that time, but that they did know that less insulin was associated with weight loss.

The frequency of using diabulimia (inducing continual hyperglycaemia and ketoacidosis) varied among the women the author has spoken to, but many of them, having had Type 1 diabetes for twenty years or more, had developed severe and chronic complications due to their previous poor diabetes self-management and this resulted in deep regret, "wishing they could turn the clock back", or "wishing I knew then what I know now." Because of changing life circumstances, such as getting married or wanting to start a family, these women had eventually stopped their diabulimic behaviour. This was not, however, as a consequence of any recognition of the disorder by the medical profession, or any medical or psychological intervention to alter this destructive action and halt the inducement of high blood glucose levels.

As seen previously with athletes taking substances to enhance their sporting performance in the short-term, the long-term consequences of certain actions on health are not a consideration at the time if the benefits are seen to outweigh any risks. However, taking enough insulin to treat hyperglycaemia in Type 1 diabetes is, of course a necessity rather than a choice, although the converse is also true in that diabulimic behaviour is also a choice. These women (the details are kept deliberately vague as requested for the purposes of anonymity) the author has discussed diabulimia with had deliberately restricted their insulin dosage repeatedly as a weight loss technique over a number of years. They had begun the practice in their early teens, paying little regard to the dangers, if indeed they were aware, of what might happen to their health in the future as a result. All of these individuals regretted their actions deeply in hindsight, and with their current knowledge of the seriousness of diabetic complications and how they can be prevented or ameliorated by maintaining good control of blood glucose levels.

In the 1970s however (when the majority of these women practised diabulimia), urine testing for glucose was the standard measure of how well diabetes was controlled, with the individual carrying out this test in the morning and before bed, and blood tests only being performed infrequently during hospital clinic visits. Now, with the widespread availability of home blood glucose meters and the use of continuous glucose sensors for those with difficult to control Type 1 diabetes, management of the condition has become very much easier. Despite this, the overwhelming desire to lose weight, coupled with potential adolescent denial of the seriousness of Type 1 diabetes, has not abated. This means that even now, diabulimia is an issue among many individuals with the condition.

In addition, the number of people with Type 1 diabetes who do not proactively manage their condition in order to achieve good diabetes control and prevent complications is, unfortunately, high. Denial of the seriousness of Type 1 diabetes and its consequences has been associated with disordered eating in young females with this chronic condition, where a significant non-concordance (deciding not to follow an agreed diabetes care plan) in sticking to a diabetes regime was shown to be accompanied by the development of microvascular (small blood vessels) complications (Goebel-Fabbri et al, 2008).

Because weight loss using the method of induced ketoacidosis is not permanent once the prescribed insulin dosage is resumed, the practice of diabulimia becomes ultimately pointless but obsessively addictive and is ongoing because the demands of diabetes are always there with the temptation to misuse insulin again and again. All of the women who have discussed this subject with the author stated that, at the time, they did not know how dangerous inducing ketoacidosis was in terms of the condition being classed as a serious medical emergency and that they were unaware of what they were doing to their bodies.

One woman who had practised diabulimia from the age of 15 stated that, at the time, she thought she was very lucky as she had a technique of losing weight very quickly that her friends did not have. She felt it was the one positive aspect of having Type 1 diabetes and by taking only a few units of insulin for two or three days, she was able to lose up to a stone (14 pounds) in one week. As previously mentioned, continued hyperglycaemia eventually develops into a state of acidity due to the breakdown of fats as an alternative source of energy to glucose that cannot be easily metabolised in the lack of insulin. This results in acid by-products which, in large quantities, become an emergency situation. This woman stated that she was very careful not to reach this stage where vomiting occurs (not induced vomiting) as the body attempts to right the acidity balance, resulting in dehydration. This woman thereby achieved regular weight loss (on a monthly basis) in this way, concealing the fact from her parents, and avoiding hospitalisation for over seven years.

Twenty years after this woman first practised diabulimia, she had hypertension (high blood pressure); damage to the autonomic nerves controlling involuntary functions such as digestion and cardiac functions (autonomic neuropathy); and pronounced diabetic eye disease (retinopathy), meaning she had significant sight impairment, all of which she attributed to her recurrent diabulimia resulting in years of poor diabetes control. This woman eventually stopped her diabulimic behaviour when she got married and wanted to have children, although her diabetes consultant had stated that pregnancy was inadvisable with her volatile health status. In addition, this woman's blood glucose control was now severely affected by autonomic neuropathy affecting nerves controlling digestion, where she had developed a very slow rate of stomach emptying (a condition known as gastroparesis).

This means that after meals, insulin has to be delayed until blood glucose levels begin to rise (assessed by finger-prick blood tests). Once this occurs, insulin is then introduced in very small and regular dosages of a few units at a time by insulin pump (a method of delivering measured dosages of insulin under the skin at the rate required) because there is little food for it to act upon, taking, in this woman's case, over five hours to digest even a small meal. This condition also results in unexpected hyperglycaemia because it is very difficult to match insulin dosages to digestion rates. Ironically then, this woman's actions in deliberately inducing poor blood glucose control during diabulimia have led to a severe complication of diabetes where good control is very difficult to attain, despite her now extreme vigilance with frequent blood glucose monitoring.

People with diabetes and renal (kidney) disease also experience an associated increased risk of cardiovascular problems (Vanholder et al, 2005). Another woman with Type 1 diabetes who formerly practised diabulimia had also developed diabetic retinopathy (eye disease), kidney disease (nephropathy), and diabetic cardiomyopathy. Cardiomyopathy is a serious condition of the heart and circulatory system thought to stem from damage to the autonomic nerves controlling parts of the body not under conscious control, such as the heartbeat. This woman was extremely regretful about her diabulimia, which commenced from the age of 16 and continued periodically every few months for almost five years.

In addition to omitting her insulin over several days each time, she would deliberately binge eat high sugar foods and drink bottles of full-sugar drinks (rather than sugar-free), driven by the thirst of hypergly-caemia. This only served to introduce even more glucose into her system which worsened and quickened the onset of ketoacidosis and vomiting. Her diabetes control was (unsurprisingly) very erratic as a result and she was frequently hospitalised as a medical emergency in her teens due to repeated vomiting from ketoacidosis, leading to dehydration and circulatory system collapse. The episodes of ketoacidosis were put down to adolescent hormonal variations making her Type 1 diabetes very difficult to control, therefore requiring more and more insulin.

This woman knew that her secret actions were the cause of her repeated ketoacidosis, but felt she could not stop this behaviour because the weight loss achieved was so dramatic and noticeable. There was no particular reason for doing this that she could remember (for example, no family problems or weight issues as this was normal for her height at 9 stones, or 126 pounds), other than that she hated her diabetes. She had great difficulty coming to terms with diabetes, and felt secretly pleased that she was able to manipulate her illness in this way. This behaviour was also a means of controlling not only her weight, but also her life as a punishment to her body which had let her down by "giving her diabetes". However, repeated and severe ketoacidosis resulted in heart, kidney and eye complications for this individual due to very poor diabetes control over a number of years, something which this woman found very difficult to come to terms with having done to herself.

Shaw and Cummings (2005) have stated that the chronic complications of diabetes may take up to ten years to appear after a prolonged period of hyperglycaemia and poor diabetes control. Both of the women previously mentioned had had many years to look back on their earlier reckless behaviour in adolescence and, as a consequence, were ultimately dealing with serious diabetic complications which were either triggered by poor blood glucose control or were made much worse when they did eventually develop in persons with severely altered metabolic control. This fact was confirmed by the diabetes specialists respectively treating these women. Both women commented that confessing their previous dangerous behaviour to their diabetes health professional made them feel guilty, humiliated, stupid, regretful, angry and sad. There was the perception that they were being told off for being naughty by the specialists, with the air of, "What do you expect?", or, "You should have known better", in the context of their complications. The association between diabulimia and feelings of shame, embarrassment, a negative body image, low self-esteem, depression and anxiety has also been reported by Larranaga et al (2011).

Serious changes to the feet in people with diabetes due to neuropathy (damage to the central or peripheral nerves, or both) are common, possibly as high as 30 percent in the UK (Sidaway and Curry, 1991; Tappin et al, 1980). This is a condition that is inextricably linked with high blood glucose levels and can manifest as nerve damage or damage to the blood vessels supplying the lower legs and feet, making healing slow and leading to ulceration and possibly gangrene and amputation if the blood supply is severely impaired. This was the case for a woman who regularly contracted infections (colds, chest infections, and bladder infections due to an impaired immune system with both Type 1 diabetes and asthma) as an adolescent, causing high blood glucose levels. However, she would also deliberately exacerbate the effects of the infection-induced hyperglycaemia, and the length of the illness, by under-dosing on her insulin at the same time. This was because the illness could then be blamed for the weight loss she achieved as it had "upset her diabetes".

Although this individual was unaware of the increased need for insulin during illness, she had noticed that the less insulin she took when suffering from an infection, the worse she felt. She would drink vast quantities of water and would urinate more often: classic symptoms of severe hyperglycaemia, with resulting ketoacidosis and rapid weight loss. The woman stated that as a girl she had secretly enjoyed this, welcoming every infection as an opportunity for weight reduction by deliberately reducing insulin when her requirements were drastically increased whilst fighting infection. She was, however, actually underweight at this time (weighing just under 7 stone, or 96 pounds) and medical professionals and her mother would comment on the fact that she could not afford to lose any more weight whenever a new infection presented.

In her later teens this woman developed regular flashing pains and a hot prickling or tingling sensation in both her feet and legs, to such an extent that she often could not bear to walk on them. One morning, in her early twenties (mid-1980s), the young woman woke and found that one of her feet was extremely swollen. Instead of reporting this to her diabetes nurse or GP, she continued to hobble around on it and persisted in going to work rather than resting it, not connecting the problem with her erratic diabetes control. When the swelling eventually subsided after 14 months, she had developed severe arthritic changes as a result of diabetic neuropathy. Her big toe was completely dislocated (a condition known as hallux rigidus) and she could not feel anything, the whole toe being completely numb. Two of her other toes had also altered shape and the whole foot had spread out so that it was much wider than the other across the bridge.

When she eventually saw a diabetes specialist and let him examine her foot, she had no ankle reflexes, no awareness of external sensation such as pain (from a sharp prick test) or hot or cold. The sole of the foot had developed a large pressure point of thickened skin which threatened to ulcerate at a point corresponding to the joints of the two arthritic toes, and this damage was attributed definitively to long periods of very poor diabetes control. The diabetes consultant diagnosed this damage as a Charcot foot, a chronic complication of diabetes which refers to the degeneration of the joints of the foot due to nerve damage, loss of sensation, and excess areas of pressure. This woman could not then walk without a stick, and had to have her shoes specially made, amputation of her lower leg only being narrowly avoided.

This woman's practice of diabulimia stopped because her general health improved as she grew older, whereby she contracted fewer infections which mean her insulin needs became more stabilised, with fewer episodes of hyperglycaemia and ketoacidosis. Another key reason for ceasing her diabulimia may have been that she moved out of her childhood home and therefore had to be independent, with no sympathy or constant attention from a worried mother for their offspring during illness. However, the woman admitted that she still did not eat properly, but did now take her insulin regularly.

Another woman in her mid-thirties in a similar position had been told that the current damage to her heart and circulatory system and to her eyes was caused by her repeated episodes of ketoacidosis as a consequence of continual diabulimia in her youth. There was also some ketoacidosis due to severe infection requiring hospitalisation as an adult. Her diabetes specialist confirmed that her heart condition was so serious that she would undoubtedly die prematurely, even though she now maintained very good control of her blood glucose levels. This woman had only stopped her diabulimic behaviour when she secured a job she really enjoyed in her mid-twenties and began to feel happy with her life.

End Stage Renal Disease (E.S.R.D.) had developed in a further former diabulimia sufferer who was in her late twenties. Because her Type 1 diabetes had always been very poorly controlled from diagnosis at the age of eight years, she had adopted a fatalistic attitude to the secondary chronic complications of the condition: "they were bound to happen anyway". Microalbuminuria or small quantities of albumin protein present in the urine (albumin being the smallest and most abundant of the plasma proteins) is the first detectable sign of kidney disease, and is estimated to be present in 16–28 percent of people with diabetes (de Jong et al, 2003; Jones et al, 2002). This is due to abnormally high blood glucose levels, where glucose spills over into the urine when blood levels reach 10mmol/l (180 mg/dl) or higher. Diabetic nephropathy, or renal disease, is defined as a persistent and clinically detectable level of protein in the urine in association with an elevated blood pressure and reduced kidney function (MacIssacs and Watts, 2005).

Because poorly-controlled diabetes causes damage to the kidney tissue, both Type 1 and Type 2 diabetes are currently the leading cause of end-stage kidney disease in Western countries. As a result of severe diabetic kidney disease, this woman was awaiting a kidney transplant and was undergoing regular dialysis. This individual ceased practising diabulimia because she felt tired and had no energy for the period leading up to when serious kidney disease was diagnosed. She reasoned that the onset of ketoacidosis would only make her feel worse and, once she received the diagnosis of kidney failure, weight loss then ceased to be a priority.

A now middle-aged woman who had practised diabulimia in her adolescence and early twenties, but not regularly (meaning four times over a period of seven years, each requiring hospitalisation), was also stoical, feeling that diabetes leads to complications sooner or later, even if it is well controlled. This view, of course, absolves the individual from any responsibility of having caused or contributed to their complications due to deliberate insulin omission or under-dosing. This was also the case for a token male who, as a middle-aged adult rather than as an adolescent female with Type 1 diabetes, admitted to sometimes "binge eating and not taking his insulin properly" (meaning missing injections), and also that he had noticed that this helped him keep his weight down.

However, this did not appear to be the same behaviour or mind set as the absolute determination of the women to deliberately lose weight with severe ketoacidosis as a consequence, although any weight loss in this man's case was also as a result of poor diabetes control. This highlights the issue of ignorance of the effects of high blood glucose levels and not monitoring insulin needs correctly, and whether this is the same thing psychologically as deliberately omitting insulin with the intention that extreme weight loss occurs. This man had also developed a number of chronic complications (eye disease, nerve damage, kidney disease, and heart disease) after having Type 1 diabetes for over 30 years, but he felt that this was just part of having the condition rather than due to his repeated hyperglycaemia and elevated HbA1c level.

It could be said that, with ongoing diabetes education about the effects of high blood glucose levels over time, this man and the women previously discussed would have been more aware of the damage being caused to their bodies. This would mean that these individuals could make an informed choice regarding their health actions. Could the knowledge that devastating complications severely affect quality of life have altered their insulin omission decisions? There is a school of thought which states that the altered metabolic parameters in diabetes mean that it is difficult, if not practically impossible, to rectify this imbalance, even if the person with diabetes attains perfect control of their condition at all times. In reality, this is rarely achievable with constant natural and unexplained fluctuations in blood glucose levels from diagnosis, and with disruption to blood glucose levels with illnesses, stress, hormonal variations and life-changing events affecting diabetes control for women, such as pregnancy.

The author has been told by her own diabetes care team that complications are inevitable eventually in every person with the condition. Therefore, there is little doubt that abnormally high blood glucose levels over a period time (as opposed to infrequent or one-off high results) do lead to the development of serious complications, as seen by these examples, and as demonstrated unequivocally by the Diabetes Control and Complications Trial (1993; 1995).

## UNDERSTANDING BEHAVIOURAL CHANGE

Knowing the risks of high blood glucose levels by providing (health professionals) or accessing (the individual) information does not lead to behavioural change on its own. This is an incredibly complex subject which involves the individual wanting to alter their damaging health behaviour because they perceive a risk in not doing so. This entails the individual recognising a threat to their health status; then considering if they will take appropriate action; then deciding when to take that action and what action this will be; then implementing the change in their behaviour for a sustained period, which may even return to the original unhealthy behaviour in a cyclical process. This is known as The Stages of Change model, first proposed by Prochaska and DiClemente (1984), and applied to addictive behaviours. Certain aspects of the model have been examined in order to understand the process of behaviour change associated with various health behaviours, including diabetes self-care. The main stages of this model are pre-contemplation of change, where the individual has not considered changing their behaviour; contemplation, where the individual becomes aware of the benefits of change and may seek information and advice in order to make an informed decision; planning, where the individual views the proposed change as both possible and worthwhile; action, where the individual makes a sustained commitment to change their behaviour; and maintenance, where the individual sustains the healthy behaviour for longer than six months (Prochaska and DiClemente, 1984; Wilson, 2009).

The Stages of Change model is suited to addictive behaviours, such as diabulimia, because it allows for relapse then a return to the contemplation phase again in a cyclical rather than a linear fashion. As diabulimia is a secretive condition where the individual may frequently return to unhealthy behaviour which can be triggered after a number of months, relapse is likely. However, in order to overcome the disorder, the individual must decide that they will not omit or reduce their insulin purposefully and that weight loss with this method is dangerous and is not permanent, meaning there is a likelihood of the individual becoming stuck at the relapse and contemplation phases rather than moving on to the action (stopping the practice of insulin under-dosing) and maintenance (taking responsibility to manage diabetes effectively) phases. Katz and Perberdy (1995) have argued that behaviour is firmly rooted within the individual's social and cultural environments so therefore, the circumstances of the person's life can make changing their behaviour very difficult. This again highlights the possible reasons for diabulimic behaviour: failure to accept the diagnosis of Type 1 diabetes and its disease management demands; weight gain as insulin treatment commences and an over-emphasis on food as part of the diabetes management regime; dysfunction within the family due to the diagnosis of diabetes and the changes which must occur to incorporate it into daily routine; coping with adolescence; continual peer pressure to be thin; and any other issues which may be present in that individual's life.

A further model used to understand health behaviour is the Health Belief model (Becker, 1974), although this was originally proposed to predict protective health behaviours such as taking up the opportunity of screening and vaccinations. The Health Belief model suggests that in order for an individual to recognise that they are engaging in unhealthy behaviour, they must first acknowledge that they are susceptible to a particular disease and its complications, and that any preventative action will have a positive effect before they can attempt to make a change. The individual must then decide to weigh up the pros and cons of changing their particular behaviour, in this case, diabulimia.

Risk prevention is therefore key to the role of certain beliefs in stimulating preventative behaviour: the individual must realise the dangers of diabulimia and decide to cease the behaviour in order to prevent future complications from arising. This is far easier said than done. As previously mentioned, short-term benefits of weight loss outweigh any future risks of developing chronic complications in the early years of living with Type 1 diabetes. Dishman (1968) identified four main disincentives to improving health-related behaviour: effort, time, health limitations, and obstacles. These obstacles were likely to be the individual's own reasons for not changing their behaviour, rather than explanations for it.

In addition to the complexities of diabulimia, a further concept of self-efficacy in health behaviour has been suggested, so that the individual believes that they are capable of adopting a positive change (Bandura, 1977). In terms of addressing and treating diabulimia, it can be seen that the individual must play the pivotal role in recognising the dangers of this behaviour and that they must want to stop this practice. This takes both time and effort, as well as the individual's own risk perception of chronic complications if no symptoms are currently present, making this aspect seem less important. Furthermore, this model of health behaviour is centred in compliance, or the patient doing what they are told, rather than in the current patient-centred approach.

The motivating factor, or belief system, associated with the Health Belief model is the influence of social pressure on behaviour, such as conforming to peer group norms (Katz and Peberdy, 1997). This means that beliefs affecting health decisions may lead to poor health behaviour, describing the peer pressure faced by adolescent girls regarding their weight and disordered eating as a result. When applying this model to 24 different health conditions it has been shown that the strongest predictor of health behaviour was perceived barriers to changing that particular behaviour and perceived susceptibility to the condition [chronic complications] in question (Janz and Becker, 1984). However, rather than perceived susceptibility, knowledge has been found to be the overriding reason why, for example, women attended a cervical screening appointment (Gregory and McKie, 1991).

A lack of knowledge about health risks has also been found to be the main reason why women did not attend screening appointments: because they did not think they had any symptoms (Harlan et al, 1991). The same has been seen regarding breast cancer screening, where factors such as family history of the disease (actual risk) and vulnerability (perceived risk) were the reasons for attending screening appointments (McCaul et al, 1996).Therefore, it is rare that all the factors of the Health Belief model are the reason why an individual decides to take positive action about their health. In terms of diabetes self-care however, (as no qualitative studies were found specifically examining diabulimia and the reasons why suffers stop this unhealthy behaviour), knowledge of and perceived risk of chronic complications prior to their development has been shown not to alter behaviour (Golin et al, 2001; Day, 1995; Donovan and Blake, 1992).

It has been found that the Health Belief model does not predict who will and who will not take on certain aspects of their diabetes self-care, such as regularly testing blood glucose levels, or taking the correct insulin dosages (Glasgow et al, 1999; Stabler et al, 1988). In addition, certain behaviours, such as taking exercise or adhering to a prescribed diet were not undertaken whilst simultaneously carrying out regular blood tests, showing that individuals do not have an "all or nothing" approach, but will undertake certain positive health behaviours if they want to, or see a benefit in doing so. A difference was also seen in those with long-duration diabetes and complications, where this meant more self-care than in the newly-diagnosed.

It appears then that different variables are more prominent to certain health behaviours and take precedence at different times in the life of a person with diabetes according to their priorities; for example, weight loss at whatever cost for an adolescent female with a strong awareness of self-image, or regular blood glucose testing for a middle-aged individual with Type 1 diabetes and complications. Both the Health Belief model and the Stages of Change model assume that the individual analyses their behaviour in terms of the good and bad aspects, weighing up the pros and cons of continuing the behaviour or not, then deciding whether to change it based on this outcome. This is probably unlikely for most people and even more so for adolescent females, with all that this entails, trying to cope with a chronic health condition.

It is not only the attitudes and health beliefs of adolescents with Type 1 diabetes and diabulimia that are relevant in recognising the important aspects that contribute to diabetes self-care. General practitioners have been found to have a far bleaker outlook concerning people with diabetes than hospital doctors, believing that the disease carries many risks, such as ketoacidosis and chronic complications, meaning that they had a lower confidence in achieving treatment goals (Marteau and Kinmouth, 1988). Because of these beliefs this study showed that GPs allowed their patients to have a wider range of blood glucose levels (meaning higher than the normal range), although this study was prior to the confirmation in 1993 that high blood glucose concentrations lead to the development of chronic complications. In terms of adolescent females with diabulimia however, this research implies that control of blood glucose levels may not be the priority, as health professionals are often at a loss regarding how to motivate behaviour change when insulin is being deliberately omitted.

Other studies, concerning the development of a diabetes attitude scale for health professionals, have shown that the negative attitudes, beliefs, and assumptions (rather than facts) of health professionals from all disciplines, especially dieticians, about the way people manage this chronic condition had detrimental effects on the individual's diabetes self-care efforts (Rossing et al, 2001; Anderson et al, 1989; 1987). This clearly has a bearing on the health behaviour of adolescents with Type 1 diabetes, deliberately mis-managing their condition to lose weight, if they perceive that their health professional [dietician] is judging them. However, the latter two studies of health professionals' attitudes were also conducted before the Diabetes Control and Complications Trial (1993; 1995) which may have had a bearing on responses, although the 1989 and 1987 studies supported active diabetes management, showing negative attitudes concerning patients who did not maintain good control of their blood glucose levels, leading to complications.

## HELPING SUFFERERS OVERCOME DIABULIMIA

Shaban (2013) has stated that as many as one-third of people with Type 1 diabetes, predominantly adolescent females and young women, practice diabulimia. Frequent admission to hospital to treat diabetic ketoacidosis is not only an important issue because of the considerable cost of providing health care, but also in terms of a reduced quality of life for the individual. The National Diabetes Inpatient Audit (2011) and the National Paediatric Audit (2011) showed that there were 8,472 hospital admissions concerning diabetic ketoacidosis, the highest incidence being among 10–19 year-old mostly female patients. This figure correlates with a 16 percent increase in admissions for eating disorders when compared to the previous year, more than half of which were in the same age range (Health and Social Care Information Centre, 2012; Shaban, 2013).

Practising diabulimia is damaging to long-term health, but in the short-term, may also become a dangerous exercise which is adopted when there are problems in the individual's life, such as family disharmony, exam pressures, or even coping with Type 1 diabetes itself as an adolescent. It may be difficult for diabetes healthcare professionals to spot the signs of diabulimic behaviour, but repeated episodes of severe diabetic ketoacidosis are one key sign. This manifests as poor blood glucose control because of self-induced hyperglycaemia with little or no insulin, although erratic diabetes control may also be due to infection or hormonal variations in adolescence. Psychological counselling may be considered for adolescents with continual episodes of ketoacidosis in order to understand the reasons for insulin restriction and, if appropriate, support for healthy weight loss should be offered to the individual. However, in the UK, diabetes services do not usually have a counsellor of clinical psychologist attached to the team due to availability on the National Health Service, making it more difficult to access treatments, such as cognitive behavioural therapy (CBT), which can help overcome destructive behaviour patterns.

Clearly the individual practising diabulimia will need to confess this behaviour and be assured that they trust and can communicate with the person or team offering them help. This may be very difficult if the person is not ready to admit to diabulimia, as it is a very secretive behaviour. If it is openly discussed, the individual must not perceive that they are being judged or blamed for their behaviour, as this is counterproductive. A study of health professional's attitudes towards adolescents with Type 1 diabetes who also had an eating disorder found that discussion of eating behaviour and weight control was only forthcoming if a rapport had been built up between patient and professional, highlighting the need for communication skills in this area (Tierney et al, 2008).

The women who have discussed diabulimia with the author have stated that it was difficult to speak to health professionals because a different staff member tended to be in the diabetes clinic every time they visited; and that the attitudes of health professionals tended to be judgemental and blaming if they had poor diabetes control and weight management issues. This meant that the women would avoid going to their diabetes clinic appointments if at all possible, making the issue of identifying disordered eating and seeking help even more difficult. It has been suggested that diabetes education alone is inadequate in addressing the problem of diabulimia as it is a complex psychological issue (Shaban, 2013). Even with help from a clinical psychologist or counsellor, and diabetes education regarding the dangers of diabulimia in terms of poor diabetes self-management and the development of chronic complications, those individuals determined to use diabulimia to lose weight will find it incredibly hard to alter their behaviour.

In these times where the Internet is frequently turned to for health advice, it would seem appropriate that diabulimia sufferers would be able to seek support in this way, also allowing them to remain anonymous. The National Health Service is increasingly using technology to communicate with patients, such as using text messaging of test result information. This has been shown to be particularly useful in communicating with hard to reach groups such as teenagers with Type 1 diabetes (Cole-Lewis and Kershaw, 2010). Access to information and support is especially necessary when the condition is not medically recognised as a problem for adolescents (or older females and males) with Type 1 diabetes, so there are no diabetes centres with specific expertise in this area. However, there is only patchy advice and support available for diabulimia sufferers to access via the Internet.

Unfortunately, the American Diabetes Association (www.diabetes.org) did not provide any information or links to diabulimia on their website at the time of access by the author. Neither did The Behavioural Diabetes Institute (www.behaviouraldiabetesinstitute.org), who failed to recognise diabulimia as a condition affecting those with Type 1 diabetes. This was also the case with psychiatric and psychological websites such as The American Psychiatric Association (www.psych.org) and The American Psychological Association (www.apa.org).

Diabetes UK (www.diabetes.org.uk) did however mention diabulimia on their website, giving a definition of both the disorder and other recognisable eating disorders; the name (although not the full contact details) of a Professor of psychology who has a special interest in diabulimia and who is affiliated to Diabetes UK; and their response to the growing incidence of the condition. Their press release has stated that one in three young women is now affected by diabulimia, highlighting the dangers of this practice, and complications which arise from high blood glucose levels. The Juvenile Diabetes Research Foundation (JDRF) (www.jdrf.org) acknowledged diabulimia as a condition and offered a support team for young people with Type 1 diabetes on their website. The National Eating Disorders Association (www.nationaleatingdisorders.org) also provided a definition of the disorder and links to a diabulimia helpline.

As technological means are becoming a more and more popular way to deliver health information and support for a number of health conditions, and this has been shown to be an effective way to communicate with young people with diabetes, the availability and provision of diabulimia support on the Internet being a way of connecting. However, it may be the case that a diabulimia sufferer, seeking support for this complex and potentially deadly disorder, feels even more isolated and alone when they find that their eating disorder is not recognised by the medical profession, and is completely overlooked or barely mentioned by certain diabetes or psychological websites.

Because diabulimia is not a recognised eating disorder in its own right, many psychologists and those treating eating disorders do not have the experience necessary to understand the condition and effectively treat someone suffering from it (Tierney et al, 2008). What is necessary in cases of diabulimia is an in-depth psychological evaluation of the individual in order for an assessment to be made of their mental health status (Hasken et al, 2010). Psychological evaluation by an expert in this area (not a diabetes nurse who may feel unequipped to deal with such a sensitive and complex issue of diabetes care) is essential for the detection of mental health states such as depression, linked to diabulimia, which adversely affects diabetes self-care, and is extremely prevalent; depression being seen in one in five people with diabetes (Kelly et al, 2005).

Depression interacts negatively with diabetes (Clark, 2003), leading to erratic diabetes control and a 1.8 percent increase in HbA1c (Mazze et al, 1984) meaning that depression has been directly linked to the development of chronic complications (Anderson et al, 2001; Lustman et al, 2000; Talbot and Nouwen, 2000). Dietary restrictions imposed by a diabetes regime and weight gain as a consequence of insulin treatment are both risk factors in the development of eating disorders such as diabulimia. Colton et al (2007) have pointed out that this presents a dilemma for clinicians attempting to treat individuals with Type 1 diabetes and diabulimia as attempts to encourage weight maintenance within normal range may lead to the individual reacting by overeating and binge eating, whilst failing to address body weight, meaning this is equally unconducive to health.

It has been suggested that regular screening of weight and eating behaviour is one way to tackle disordered eating in those with diabetes, focussing on "normal" eating and increased self-esteem (Colton et al, 2007). However, in the author's experience, this would lead to deliberate avoidance of appointments as this kind of intervention only serves to highlight the subject of weight and food even more, rather than directly tackling the reasons why disordered eating and insulin omission occur, such as family problems, depression, and self-destruction as a punishment for a body that has "let the individual down", which may not be related to low self-esteem.

Many things disrupt control of blood glucose levels, meaning a rise above the recommended maximum 7mmol (l126mg/dl). In order to realise this however, the individual with Type 1 diabetes is advised to check their blood glucose levels 4–6 times a day and even more frequently if exercising or during illness. Because diabulimia is effectively ignoring the fact that insulin is required and that Type 1 diabetes is a chronic and serious disease that must be managed in order to avoid or slow the onset of complications, blood glucose levels are not tested regularly, if at all. The issue that needs to be addressed by health professionals is therefore termed as non-concordance, or the refusal of a person with diabetes to work with their diabetes team to achieve the best possible control of the disease.

Diabulimia is a secretive and self-destructive process and many excuses will be made rather than admitting to the truth. Because hormonal variations, puberty, food, stress, emotional upset, exercise, and illness can all dramatically effect blood glucose levels, even if the individual is really trying to control these continual fluctuations, these reasons can also be used as an excuse for poor control in diabulimia, as seen by some of the previous examples. From personal experience of someone who was in denial about their diabetes from diagnosis to her early twenties, it does not matter what health professionals tell you time and time again, or the grisly pictures of amputated limbs and gangrenous sores because of diabetes which are shown to you (as mentioned, these have stayed with me but did not have the desired effect until many years later), a change in behaviour will only occur when the individual is ready to acknowledge the seriousness and consequences of the disease.

There is clearly difficulty in firstly recognising the condition of diabulimia (the individual admitting to themselves that they have a problem) and the individual being able to access appropriate help from heath professionals with a good knowledge of the condition and effective strategies to offer. There is sporadic assistance available to diabulimia suffers online (especially in the US) and few research studies have been undertaken to assess the various approaches used to treat eating disorders (Criego and Jahraus, 2009), especially so because diabulimia is not fully recognised as a problem. In addition, once adolescents move to an adult diabetes clinic at age 18, this can be traumatic necessitating a change in consultant, nurse and familiar faces (Wilson, 2010).

Collaboration between the diabetes team and psychological support is necessary and essential to address this potentially life-threatening behaviour. Shaban (2013) has stated that eating disorders can be successfully treated and diabetes can be optimally managed with the adoption of a multidisciplinary approach, adding that diabetes teams need to have a high level of suspicion for the presence of an eating disorder before asking questions. However, the individual may only visit their diabetes care team once or twice a year, and if diabulimia is being practiced, that person may skip appointments altogether because poor blood glucose control will be highlighted.

In the first instance, the individual must recognise that they have a problem with deliberate insulin under-dosing and then be able to trust their diabetes health professional in order to admit to this. This will continue to be an issue until the individual is ready to address their diabulimia, where hormonal variations and infection or emotional upset will continue to be blamed for erratic diabetes self-management until readiness for change is reached. It may, sadly, only be the onset of chronic complications that act as a trigger to cease diabulimia and poor diabetes control. However, before reaching this ultimate stage of complications, vigilance by parents and health professionals regarding how frequently blood glucose testing strips, lancets and insulin are being re-ordered on prescription is a very good indicator that an individual's diabetes is not being monitored or self-managed correctly.

# CHAPTER FIVE

# INSULIN AS A MURDER WEAPON

A large enough dose of insulin can kill. However, this relies on the size of the individual and whether they have any underlying heath conditions that make them more vulnerable. It is rare that an individual will die form the single factor of an insulin overdose, or hypoglycaemia. Brain damage and eventual death will result if the blood glucose level is too low to sustain brain function, but this can possibly take days (Marks and Richmond, 2007). There will be an increase in adrenaline accompanying a low blood glucose level which can lead to multiple organ failure and an altered cardiac rhythm (cardiac arrhythmia). Deliberate and accidental overdoses of insulin are far more common than one would expect; the first case of suicide using insulin occurred in 1927, and by 1963 a total of 13 other cases of death known to be due to insulin overdose had been recorded (Marks and Richmond, 2007).

Worryingly, the people we expect to care for us when we are ill are often the perpetrators of a suspicious insulin death, giving rise to headlines claiming that insulin has been used as a poison by health professionals to kill. However, insulin is not a poisonous substance to body tissues. As with the use of insulin in sport, attempted murder using insulin is thought to be the perfect crime because insulin is naturally produced by the body, disappearing very quickly without trace, and therefore making it difficult to identify at post mortem. This is, of course, not normally the case with modern-day forensic methods and mass spectrometry testing, able to detect even minute samples of insulin in human tissue. However, until fairly recently, death by insulin causing severe hypoglycaemia relied upon the interpretation and knowledge of insulin experts as the validity of laboratory results was often flawed (Marks, 1993).

Although accidental hypoglycaemia is rarely the cause of death, deliberately induced hypoglycaemia is far more often deadly. Fortunately, the body has a mechanism to counteract the effects of plummeting blood glucose levels, whereby the liver releases stored glycogen; and glycogenolysis occurs; a process accelerated by glycogen where stored glucose in the liver is converted into usable glucose to raise blood glucose levels. As previously mentioned, the symptoms of severe hypoglycaemia are dramatic and cause immense confusion, disorientation, emotional anguish, anxiety, fear, and panic in the sufferer. For this reason, hypoglycaemia has been cited as the most-feared of diabetic complications (McCrimmon and Frier, 1994).

Whilst severe hypoglycaemia can be detected with blood testing in life, blood glucose levels after death are not the same, and hypoglycaemia is difficult to determine as an exact cause of death (Marks, 2006). It was considered that the detection of insulin as a murder weapon would be easier to solve once a suitable blood test was developed (Marks and Richmond, 2007), although this is not always the case. Insulin is detectable in both the blood and urine of a dead body, and this can be an indication of foul play. Many of the following reported cases also appear in far more forensic and descriptive detail in Marks and Richmond's brilliant book, *Insulin Murders: True Life Cases* (2007).

## THE FIRST INSULIN MURDER

In Bradford, Yorkshire on the afternoon of May 4, 1957, a 32-year old woman, Elizabeth Barlow, lay in her bath. Her husband, Kenneth, had found her seemingly unconscious late the night before. Kenneth, a state-registered nurse, claimed Elizabeth had gone to bed early, but had felt sick and hot, sweating profusely, and had decided to have a bath. Her husband had fallen asleep in his wife's absence and, waking later, realised that she was still in the bath at 11:20pm. In the bathroom he found Elizabeth's body had sunk beneath the water but that he could not lift her. In desperation he held her head above water whilst draining the bath, attempting ineffectual artificial respiration (the method he later described was not correct to try and induce breathing). Kenneth then called the family doctor who swiftly arrived and confirmed that Elizabeth was dead. They had been married less than a year.

Because the death was unexpected the police were called, along with the on-call Home Office forensic pathologist. The pathologist declared that this was an unnatural death because it was highly unlikely for a previously healthy young woman to die in her bath tub. He also noted that there was the equivalent to a small cupful of water residing between the bend of Elizabeth's arm and the side of the bath, making her husband's resuscitation story highly unlikely. The evidence mounted as the police found two used syringes in the Barlow's home, although a search for injectable substances such as insulin drew a blank.

A post mortem examination was conducted six hours after death. This showed that Elizabeth's pupils were widely dilated and that her nose, mouth and throat contained blood-stained froth (Birkinshaw et al, 1958). Her lungs were congested and haemorrhaged, consistent with death by drowning. Sadly it was found that Elizabeth had been eight weeks pregnant when she died. The pathologist took numerous blood samples from different areas of the body, and a urine sample, convinced that Elizabeth had been unconscious prior to her drowning. He also suspected that she had been injected with insulin. The symptoms of hypoglycaemia

Elizabeth had experienced: feeling hot, profuse sweating, and sickness, described by Kenneth Barlow; and the finding that Elizabeth's pupils were widely dilated, certainly pointed towards this conclusion.

Four days later Elizabeth's body underwent a further, more extensive, examination and two injection marks were discovered, one on each buttock. Tissue samples of these injection sites were removed and stored for insulin testing, rarely available at the time. A laboratory able to carry out such as test was located. Marks and Richmond (2007) have stated that at this time, these tests relied on detecting the dose of insulin that caused hypoglycaemic convulsions in mice, and then comparing this to standardised samples containing measured amounts of insulin to determine the correct concentration. By July 5, the results of the insulin sample tests were received. A total of 84 units of insulin had been found in the tissues of the buttocks (Marks and Richmond, 2008a); a hefty dose for any person with diabetes, although Elizabeth Barlow did not have the condition.

Twenty-one days later the police questioned Kenneth Barlow and an admission was made of injection of an illegal abortion-inducing drug (ergometrine), an exercise that Elizabeth was apparently fully complicit with. This was not supported by the evidence found during the drug tests carried out on Elizabeth's body, nor by the tests on the syringes and needles found in the Barlow's home. The insulin samples were again tested using the recently-available and far more sensitive method of measuring the amount of radioactive glucose taken up by the muscle tissue. After numerous different techniques were employed to rule out any false-positive results, the original findings were shown to be correct. At the trial, the prosecution deliberated whether Elizabeth could have injected herself in the buttocks with insulin, as some people chose to administer insulin for their own reasons, as seen earlier in the case of athletes, or in cases of suicide. It was decided that it is rather difficult to inject insulin into one's own buttocks, although the author has done so on many occasions to treat diabetes, delivering insulin at an alternative site to rest the abdomen, legs and arms.

Although vision of the area (buttocks) is clearly difficult, aiming the needle into the tissue is not a problem. The prosecution decided that Elizabeth must have been injected by someone else as she was unlikely to have injected insulin into her own buttocks. Kenneth Barlow had unfortunately been unable to keep his ideas to himself. It was revealed that he had boasted to his nursing colleagues a number of times that it would be very easy to murder someone using insulin as it was a substance that could not be traced. Although Elizabeth was found to have a large amount of insulin present in the test samples, which would ultimately reveal Kenneth as the perpetrator, no insulin was found in the used syringes left in the house. It is unusual to have this type of medical equipment present if there was no need for it, and one wonders why the syringes were there, although Kenneth had also injected Elizabeth with ergometrine.

Kenneth Barlow was unable to explain the presence of insulin in his wife's body at his trial in December, 1957. Adamant that he did not commit the murder, Barlow was sentenced to a 26-year prison term which he served, being released in 1984. Although insulin was present when Elizabeth was found dead, the post mortem evidence also showed that her lungs were saturated with bath water as a result of her drowning. Whilst it is not known how much insulin was actually injected, as a proportion would have been absorbed into the bloodstream and degraded, the 84 units found did not kill Elizabeth on its own, although it did lead to an unconscious state. As previously mentioned, Mrs Barlow was already suffering hypoglycaemic effects (sickness, feeling very hot and sweaty, and pupil dilation) when she went to have her bath.

As Kenneth was a nurse and claimed, even on release from prison, that he did not kill his wife, one wonders why he did not stay with her during her bath if she were ill, or even suggest that she did not have one at all? There was also no mention of whether Elizabeth was suffering from disorientation and poor co-ordination with this level of hypoglycaemia progressively getting worse. Clearly it will never be known whether Elizabeth did obtain insulin and, for whatever reason, injected it herself. However, the evidence suggests that Kenneth was the person who did this. Perhaps he encouraged her to have a bath because she was hot and this enabled him to drown her whilst she was disorientated, or indeed, unconscious from hypoglycaemia. As Marks and Richmond (2007) have stated, if it was Kenneth Barlow's intention to kill his wife, he could have encouraged her to stay in bed and succumb to death by hypoglycaemia, or at least irreversible brain damage, whereby all of the insulin would have disappeared from his wife's body leaving no case against him.

### THE INVOLVEMENT OF INSULIN IN A LOVE TRIANGLE

On the evening of the January 4, 1959, it was not a happy new year for a young woman in Bonn, Germany. This 32-year old lay dead in the home she shared with her husband. The local doctor was called after it was suggested by the husband that her death was due to heart failure caused by an over-active thyroid gland; a condition also known as thyrotoxicosis, Grave's disease, and hyperthyroidism. An excess of thyroid hormone speeds up the heart rate, causes tremor, nervousness, hyperactivity, intolerance to heat, and breathlessness because the hormone controls metabolic rate. There are instances where heart failure can occur in association with this condition, but these are rare (Krishnamoorthy et al, 2009; Valcavi et al, 1992; Rives and Shepard, 1951). Because far less was known about this disorder in the 1950s, the doctor accepted this explanation without question, certifying the death as heart failure due to thyrotoxicosis without examining the body (Marks and Richmond, 2007).

As a result, the woman's body was buried on January 7, without undergoing a post mortem. However, a suspicious relative felt that she had not died from natural causes, and the body was exhumed for examination. This revealed, among other minor injuries, numerous injection marks on the upper arms and thighs. Because of the high profile death of Elizabeth Barlow only two years before, awareness was high in case insulin had also been used in this instance, and samples were duly taken from the injection sites. These were sent to the University of Frankfurt for analysis by a diabetes expert. Again, these tests relied on detecting the dose of insulin that caused hypoglycaemic convulsions in mice, and then comparing this to standardised samples containing measured amounts of insulin to determine the correct concentration (Marks and Richmond, 2007).

When the test results were received the tissue samples were found to contain a large quantity of insulin, despite the fact that several days of insulin degradation had occurred. With this irrefutable evidence, the woman's husband and his mistress, a nurse caring for terminally-ill patients, confessed all. They had tried to remove the unwanted wife from the love triangle by several callous methods over the four days preceding her death, including extreme alcohol poisoning on New Year's Eve. This attempt was thwarted when the woman was violently sick meaning the amount of alcohol absorbed was seriously reduced. A couple of days after this she was rendered unconscious by a blow to the head, and later that same day, after recovering from the blow, she was injected intravenously with a mixture of petrol and air.

Refusing to die, even after swallowing a dose of barbiturates (sedatives which lower blood pressure, body temperature, and depress the central nervous system and respiration) also administered by the pair, the husband and his mistress attempted their final assault. Over the following two days, 400 units of insulin, stolen from the nurse's workplace, were given to the woman on three occasions, both directly into the vein, and into muscle (Marks and Richmond, 2007). A combination of the injuries sustained and the insulin dosages were what finally killed the woman demonstrating, as Marks and Richmond (2007) have stated, that insulin overdose alone is rarely the sole cause of death, and that it neither kills quickly or without trace.

## THE INSULIN SERIAL KILLER

On March 15, 1968 in America a 55-year old man with various pseudonyms was found guilty of several counts of murder following a 20-year killing spree and after dispatching two of his seven wives and his nephew (Marks and Richmond, 2007). Insulin was the weapon of choice as it was thought to be undetectable, and could still be bought over the counter in pharmacies, not becoming a prescription-only drug until 1998. This man (his true name being William Archerd), similar to the English serial killer Reginald Christie in 1953, had delusions of being a doctor but was denied the opportunity to work in this field of medicine. In 1950 an earlier transgression was uncovered whereby Archerd had been found in possession of the painkiller, morphine, receiving a 5-year probationary sentence for his crime. He was also imprisoned for a second drug-related offence, but escaped after serving only one year in 1951, being re-captured and serving a further two years in San Quentin prison (Marks and Richmond, 2007). By 1956 Archerd was living with his third wife, Zella, in Los Angeles. He reported a robbery with violence to the police where intruders had subjected the pair to injection of a substance at gunpoint, stealing a sum of money in the process. The wife duly died following her ordeal and four injection sites were found on the woman's buttocks, but suspiciously none were present on Archerd's. However, before death, police had managed to question his disorientated spouse who fully supported her husband's version of events, although she claimed she had not seen the intruders as her vision had been obscured. The police were clearly concerned at the woman's state of health having discovered a syringe in the house and a half-empty bottle of long-acting insulin outside the premises. Her level of hypoglycaemia worsened to coma and fits due to brain damage (Asvoid et al, 2010; Bree et al, 2009) and Zella died in hospital the next day. One police officer highlighted his suspicion of the insulin that was found, but this was dismissed by the coroner as insulin is not considered a poison.

On March 12, 1958, almost ten years to the day when Archerd would later be found guilty of multiple murders, his fifth wife, Juanita, was found unconscious; they had only been married for two days. She died in hospital several hours later, but this was attributed to an overdose of sedatives (although not tested). Tests were also not carried out to determine blood glucose levels, although later evidence suggested that hypoglycaemic coma contributed towards Juanita's death. Marrying for a sixth time, Archerd decided to strike a deadly blow to the head of his new spouse's ex-husband, a murder for which he escaped accountability, it being attributed to accidental causes. Because these two deaths occurred in an area of the USA (Nevada) out of the jurisdiction of the suspicious policeman involved in the death of wife number three, he could not act (Marks and Richmond, 2007). He registered his concerns with the Nevada police, but they claimed there was insufficient evidence that Archerd murdered his current wife's ex-husband; insulin overdose was also not considered.

In 1961 the Nevada newspapers reported the death of Archerd's nephew following a tragic hit-and-run road accident. Archerd had personally taken his nephew to hospital after the accident, where the younger man sustained injuries to his hip and scalp, but he also presented as semi-conscious with dilated pupils, common after head injury is sustained. Later that night, after a visit from uncle Archerd, the patient's condition worsened and he became unconscious; a state which was sustained until his death ten days later. A lumbar puncture had been performed to collect spinal fluid because of the nephew's head injury and persistent coma. This was tested and found to be low in glucose (Marks and Richmond, 2007). A post mortem was conducted and the pathologist strongly suspected that insulin had caused the comatose state, although this could not be tested because of insulin degradation and the rate that it disappears from the body (Bauman and Yalow, 1981).

Feeling certain that the nephew's accident was not the cause of death, the Los Angeles policeman, who was watching Archerd's every move, took this hit-and-run case to a colleague investigating fatal road accidents. Archerd's name was also known for motor insurance fraud after claiming for an accident which had been deliberately staged. Perhaps sensing that he had raised the suspicions of police, Archerd changed his name to James Arden. When his seventh wife, Mary had been declared bankrupt after a year of marriage, Archerd (or Arden) chose to return to his sixth wife who had escaped his murderous intentions. Although Mary survived another car accident staged by Archerd, as she was not living with him at the time, he visited her at their former home after she was released from hospital on the pretext of comforting her.

Mary was re-admitted to hospital two days later in a coma from which she did not recover; she died the next day. Blood tests were carried out and these showed a low level of blood glucose and the presence of barbiturates. Despite the fact that a very sensitive method of detecting minute amounts of insulin in tissue samples had been developed by Rosalind Yalow and Sol Berson in 1960 (Berson and Yalow, 1966), this was not employed as a test to determine if this was the cause of Mary's death (Marks and Richmond, 2007). This test has since been superseded by mass spectrometry testing as radioimmunoassay, as previously mentioned, can be subject to artefacts which hinder the authenticity of results (Mukhapadyay, 2007).

A Professor of Pathology at the University of California was asked to use his own insulin-detection techniques after being supplied with preserved post mortem samples obtained from the brain of Archerd's nephew, and samples obtained from Mary's brain. Unusually high amounts of insulin were found to be present in the tissue from both individuals. However, the expert was not sent these samples until the day Archerd's trial began on December 4, 1967, meaning that this evidence could not be used. Evidence was heard to show that Archerd had malice aforethought; that he had planned the deaths using insulin to kill his fifth wife, Juanita; the ex-husband of his sixth wife, Frank Stewart; and also a male friend, William Jones, in 1947. This last murder only came to light because of the evidence given by Archerd's second wife, who was a nurse (Marks and Richmond, 2007). However, it was alleged that William Jones allowed the injection of insulin (although completely unaware of the dangers or consequences) to appear unconscious in yet another motor insurance scam.

In his past working life, Archerd had been an attendant at the Camarillo State Mental Hospital during the period when insulin coma treatment for schizophrenia had been popular. The effects of this barbaric treatment as a result of deliberately inducing regular insulin overdose and severe hypoglycaemia for a number of hours would have been an ideal training ground regarding insulin dosages and effects for a would-be serial killer. Archerd was found guilty of three counts of first-degree murder in respect of Zella (his third wife); his nephew; and his seventh wife, Mary. He received the death sentence on March 6, 1968, but in an ironic twist, his sentence was revised to that of life imprisonment when being put to death was deemed as a "cruel and unusual punishment" by the United States Supreme Court in 1970 (Marks and Richmond, 2007). Archerd escaped being put to death, despite the re-instatement of the US Death Penalty in 1974.

Marks and Richmond (2008b) have stated that it is now know that insulin cannot accurately be detected in the brain after death as it is easily confused with other chemicals. Archerd had clearly carried out his murder spree, and his car insurance fraud, so that he would gain financially. Instead of arsenic being used as the traditional "inheritance powder", Archerd used insulin because he had witnessed its power in the case of insulin coma treatment victims. The murder of Frank Stewart, the ex-husband of Archerd's sixth wife, had occurred because of a carefully tailored plan to insure his life in the event of accident, making the beneficiaries Archerd's mother and sixth wife, although the insurance was never paid because there was insufficient evidence of accidental death (Marks and Richmond, 2007). The evidence for all-consuming greed was further supported in the case of Archerd's nephew, who had inherited a substantial compensation sum following his father's death where Archerd was the trustee of this sum, which mysteriously later disappeared. Despite Mary's bankruptcy, Archerd also stood to gain the entirety of her estate in the event of her death. Although Archerd escaped being put to death, he could not escape infection, and died from pneumonia aged 65 in 1977.

## "The Angel of Death"

In 1974, a Scottish nurse, Jessie McTavish, dubbed "The Angel of Death" by the press, was convicted of murdering a patient, 80-year old Elizabeth Lyon, with insulin. She was also charged with giving illegal injections to three other patients, although she claimed that these contained only water. McTavish received a life sentence in October 1974 but appealed against her conviction in 1975 and, in a strange twist, her lawyers successfully argued that the judge had deliberately mislead the jury by omitting the fact that McTavish had denied that this was a mercy killing (Yorker et al, 2006).

## An insulin case reaches television

Claus von Bulow was accused of attempting to murder his wife, Sunny (baptised Martha), using insulin on two occasions, and was tried in the United States courts in both 1982 and 1985. Evidence suggested he was having an affair and wished to dispose of his wife. After being found guilty in the first American trial to be televised in 1982, von Bulow was sentenced to a 30-year prison term, but an appeal in 1985 overturned this conviction due to a lack of evidence of any wrongdoing, and he was acquitted (Puccio, 1995). Sunny had inherited a generous fortune and had also been well provided for by her former marriage to a member of the nobility: an Austrian prince, Alfred von Auersperg. Sunny had also done well in her second marriage to Claus von Bulow, a very successful barrister who had partnered the late billionaire, John Paul Getty (Marks and Richmond, 2007).

After their marriage they spent their time between Sunny's two homes in New York's Fifth Avenue and Newport, Rhode Island. Clearly they were not short of wealth. Von Bulow's attorney argued that Sunny was addicted to drugs and alcohol (a charge that friends supported but that Sunny's children denied), meaning that she suffered from reactive hypoglycaemia as these substances significantly lowered her blood glucose levels. During Christmas in 1979, Sunny had entered a comatose state, being rushed as an emergency to the Newport Hospital, Rhode Island. Almost a year later she was admitted to New York's Lennox Hill hospital due to an aspirin overdose. As previously mentioned, aspirin has a glucose-lowering effect as it has the action of inhibiting the absorption of glucose in the small intestine (Arvanitikis, et al, 1977). If taken regularly, a sufficient dose of aspirin can therefore reduce blood glucose levels enough to cause frequent hypoglycaemia.

Sunny von Bulow was quickly revived following admission to Newport Hospital for her first hypoglycaemic coma in December 1979. Her husband stated that she had gone to bed without eating and after having drunk a large quantity of alcohol on December 26. The following day, Sunny felt unwell and remained in bed, occasionally drinking full-sugar soft drinks. Sunny had been very upset by the fact that her daughter planned to leave for Austria, and by the afternoon of December 27, her case worsened (Marks and Richmond, 2007). The family doctor was called and found that Sunny had difficulty breathing and was vomiting. Her breathing ceased altogether and the doctor began resuscitation as Claus von Bulow called an ambulance. Sunny's condition was attributed to oxygen depletion and inhaling her own vomit; her blood glucose level was 2.3mmol/L (41 mg/dl) and she was given an intravenous injection of glucose and a glucose drip (Marks and Richmond, 2007). No alcohol or drug traces were found in urine tests, only that of a standard dose of aspirin.

Sunny von Bulow did not regain consciousness, a blood glucose test four hours later being 1.1mmol/L (20 mg/dl) whereby she was given more glucose. She was also found to have a severe chest infection. By December

28, Sunny had recovered, but this was unlike the expected progression from an insulin coma, as brain swelling had not occurred after deep unconsciousness (Asvoid et al, 2010; Bree et al, 2009). Hypoglycaemia can also occur as a result of altered glucose metabolism in the case of severe infection, but this is rare (Marks and Richmond, 2007). Sunny was advised that an insulinoma (insulin-secreting tumour) may be the reason for her severe hypoglycaemia. It was also noted by doctors that her low blood glucose levels were probably the result of alcohol, although this was not investigated.

None of the tests carried out on Sunny revealed the cause of her hypoglycaemia. Almost one year later, Sunny's second bout of semi-consciousness and confusion was treated with glucose by paramedics, although this had no effect. However, her blood glucose level was not actually low, measured at a normal 5.7mmol/L (103mg/dl). The symptoms were later attributed to a recent head injury. Sixteen days later, on December 21, Sunny was found unconscious. She was admitted to Newport Hospital with no recordable blood pressure and an absent heartbeat. She was also suffering from hypothermia, a condition often seen with extremely low blood glucose levels (Marks and Richmond, 2007).

At the later trial it emerged that Sunny had drunk a quantity of alcohol and taken sleeping tablets the night before (Puccio, 1995). Whilst in hospital she stopped breathing and stayed on a ventilator until she was once again able to breathe for herself; however, she remained unconscious with a blood glucose level of 1.6mmol/L (29 mg/dl) which was treated with glucose. Later that evening a further test revealed that Sunny now had a high blood glucose reading of 14.4mmol/L (259mg/dl), although this became normal again without treatment by midnight but, as she was still unconscious, she was given a powerful steroid to reduce any brain swelling (Marks and Richmond, 2007).

As she had not recovered consciousness, Sunny was moved to an affiliated hospital to the Harvard Medical School; the Peter Bent Brigham Hospital, with a diagnosis of irreversible hypoglycaemic brain damage.

The initial blood sample taken showed a low blood potassium level consistent with low blood glucose levels, but this was later revealed to be due to Sunny's use of purgatives and the concentration of blood alcohol. Blood was also sent to a laboratory for glucose and insulin analysis. Because no insulin antibodies were found this was thought to be because Sunny had either been injecting insulin herself (perhaps as a weight loss technique as she also used purgatives), or because somebody else (her husband) had injected her. It was later discovered that an absence of insulin antibodies in blood is not an indication of insulin administration (Marks and Richmond, 2007).

Tests for C-peptide also indicated that levels were low; suggesting that Sunny's low blood glucose levels were due to exogenous (injected) insulin rather than any physiological cause. As previously mentioned, Claus von Bulow was then arrested for the attempted murder of his wife (Dershowitz, 1991; Wraight, 1983). In von Bulow's first trial the evidence pointed towards insulin injection by either Sunny herself, or Claus von Bulow. After the trial, von Bulow changed his legal team and this proved essential in finding him innocent, as Sunny's hypoglycaemia was shown to be due to causes other than the injection of insulin. Sunny often drank alcohol but did not eat, inducing fasting hypoglycaemia, which occurs 6–36 hours after consumption of a moderate to large amount of alcohol (Marks and Richmond, 2007). She also took sleeping pills, painkillers, sedatives and purging substances for weight loss. Her hypoglycaemic episodes and permanent comatose state were undoubtedly due to the way Sunny lived her heiress lifestyle. Sunny von Bulow remained in a vegetative state for a total of 28 years until her death on December 7, 2008.

## A DEATH-BED KILLING

A 59-year old man lay dying in the Harry Truman Veterans' Hospital in Colombia, Missouri from an incurable brain tumour. He was also a newly-wed, having only married his wife, Delores Miller, 13 days before his admission. The man, Erroll, had suffered a significant change in his personality over the two preceding months and was also suffering debilitating fits due to a brain tumour. As a result, Erroll decided to dramatically change his life, leaving his job and meeting Delores at a lonely-hearts get-together. Delores was a 52-year old nurse, so the union seemed fated. Unfortunately for Erroll, she was looking to capture her tenth husband. On February 26, 1983, Erroll's surgeon tried to remove the tumour, which had curtailed his ability to speak, but found this was not possible. Erroll and Delores were given the devastating news that he only had around six months left to live.

Six days after his surgery, Erroll lapsed into unconsciousness and stopped breathing; blood tests revealed a low blood glucose level and glucose was given, but Erroll did not recover, dying four days later (Marks and Richmond, 2007). There was nothing suspicious found at his post mortem, but since Erroll had suffered from hypoglycaemia his doctor felt this was odd, suspecting Delores of injecting her husband deliberately with insulin. Delores was closely observed from then on, and on his final day, she put on a great show of tripping over the intravenous drip equipment, throwing herself outstretched over her husband's prone body, and announcing with remarkable foresight to the attending nurse that Erroll was not long for this world. The heart monitor then showed an altered rhythm and Erroll passed away. Pre- and post-mortem blood samples revealed that Erroll had an undetectable level of blood glucose, although no insulin or C-peptide tests were performed; a high concentration of injected insulin (with no C-peptide present) was also detected in a preserved blood sample taken when Erroll first suffered hypoglycaemia (Marks and Richmond, 2007). Delores was questioned by police and she confessed to having given her husband insulin so that his condition would worsen and he would be placed in intensive care. It would seem that Delores Miller, one of the caring profession, wanted to ease her husband's suffering and perhaps even end it. However, it was revealed that Delores had taken all Erroll's savings and wagered with hospital staff that her husband would definitely die soon, having also ensured that a speedy cremation could take place.

It was now down to the prosecution to prove that Delores had caused Erroll's initial episode of hypoglycaemia. The judge, however, ruled the evidence from the blood samples inadmissible as it was difficult to confirm that the samples were original and had not been tampered with (Haibach et al, 1987). As with all hypoglycaemia deaths, insulin overdose was not the sole cause in the case of Erroll, who was terminally ill, but was a contributory factor. Marks and Richmond (2007) have surmised that Delores injected Erroll's intravenous tubing with insulin when she lay across him after pretending to stumble, the dosage causing a rapid descent in blood glucose levels [although fast-acting insulin usually takes around 20 minutes to work; this would be quicker intravenously, but not instant], triggering the release of a huge amount of adrenaline, stopping Erroll's heart. Although Delores was strongly suspected of having killed her husband with insulin, the inadmissible blood sample evidence did not help to ascertain this (Haibach et al, 1987). Her confession, although later changed, was enough to convict her of murder, and she was sentenced to life imprisonment with a stipulation that she must serve a minimum of 50 years before parole.

## A SPATE OF INFANT DEATHS

In 1991, a number of babies died in England's Grantham Hospital, Lincolnshire. The police suspected insulin overdose was the cause after this was brought to their attention on April 30. Over the past couple of months there had been an increase in the number of seriously ill children transferred from Grantham Hospital to the Queens Medical Centre in Nottinghamshire. At the same time, one of the paediatric doctors had also raised concerns about this (Askill and Sharpe, 1993). A nurse was suspended on suspicion as three babies had died unexpectedly, and possibly a fourth, with a total of 19 cases in all under examination. There was no conclusive evidence and the events leading to these deaths could have been interpreted as due to unfortunate but natural circumstances.

Samples of blood plasma had been taken from each infant and refrigerated for later testing. It was determined that nurse Beverly Allitt was the only person involved with all the patients and suspicion was strong that she was the culprit. However, opinion was divided among medical staff and poor conditions on the hospital's paediatric ward were also blamed for the increased number of deaths. One five month old baby, Paul Crampton, had been injected with a large dose of insulin on at least three occasions, but fortunately survived the experience, although a blood glucose reading of 1.0mmol/L (18mg/dl) had been recorded (Marks and Richmond, 2007). Whist this seemed to be the proof of wrongdoing that was needed, Beverly Allitt was not arrested until the beginning of September after a second baby, Becky Phillips, had died.

Despite this, the police did not charge Allitt and she was allowed to go free. Two months later, in November 1991, there was sufficient evidence to charge her with murder. Further cases were investigated up to the time Beverly was charged. A 15 month old baby, Claire Peck, was admitted to Grantham Hospital suffering from a severe asthma attack. After receiving emergency care and having recovered, the infant was left in Allitt's charge and later died. Although an excess of insulin was not found, an increased level of potassium was, so much so that the machine could not measure the amount. A fourth child, seven week old Liam Taylor, then died from cardiorespiratory arrest and, although no blood glucose levels were measured, Liam was found to have an enlarged liver, full of glycogen, consistent with him being given insulin maliciously (Marks and Richmond, 2007).

After Beverley was suspended she sought work outside the NHS. She attempted to kill a care home resident, Dorothy Lowe, with insulin, and also a 14-year old boy, Jonathan Jobson, with a blood glucose lowering drug used to treat Type 2 diabetes. At her trial there was found to be insufficient evidence to convict on these charges, but Allitt was found guilty of the murder of four children and the attempted murder of a further three, inflicting grievous bodily harm to another six. She was taken to Rampton Mental Hospital to reside there permanently until her death and 12 sets of parents were compensated for their trauma.

## SOMETHING IS AFOOT

In June 1994, Eric Lloyd died. He had been unwell for some time and was depressed after the suicide of his brother. Eric's partner Maria Whiston described how she had found Eric dead in bed on June 3 when she came home after working nights as a nurse. The family doctor certified the death and notified the police. Because his death was unexpected, a post mortem examination was arranged. Eric had a daughter, Karen, who was highly suspicious about her father's demise and felt that Maria had something to do with it. The police had found two alcohol swabs in a room, the type used to clean an area of skin before injection (Marks and Richmond, 2007). At post mortem examination bruising was found on Eric's right thigh, and it was discovered that he had an enlarged heart and blocked arteries. Samples were also taken for further testing.

On June 8, a second post mortem was conducted following Karen raising suspicion of wrongdoing. No further evidence was found that could shed any light on the reason for Eric's death, but Karen had also informed police that her father had suffered two hypoglycaemic episodes a couple of years before. In August, 1991, Eric had been admitted to his local hospital's Accident and Emergency Department in an unconscious state where it was determined that he did not have diabetes and was not prescribed insulin. He recovered after he was given glucose and, as his hypoglycaemia had no apparent cause, he was discharged a few days later. In September 1991, Eric suffered the same fate, becoming unconscious after waking with a headache. Again he was given intravenous glucose and recovered, but could not remember how he had become unwell. Eric strongly denied that he had injected himself with insulin, or that anyone else had done so (Marks and Richmond, 2007).

On his second hospital admission, Eric's blood glucose level was measured at 1.3mmol/L (23mg.dl). It also became very low, despite the glucose infusion, during his hospital stay. This was felt to be due to either an insulinoma or a deliberate injection of insulin. In the event that an insulin-secreting tumour was the cause, Eric was given a drug to prevent the secretion of insulin by his pancreas. This is only useful when there is excess insulin being produced by the patient's own body, and has no effect on fasting or reactive hypoglycaemia. For this reason, Eric continued to become hypoglycaemic, with blood samples before glucose showing the presence of a large amount of insulin, ruling out natural causes other than tumour (Marks and Richmond, 2007).

C-peptide concentration, however, was undetectable, meaning that the insulin had to have been injected rather than produced by Eric's pancreas. This meant that it was likely someone had injected Eric, although the dosages were not enough to kill on their own. Because of the repeated circumstances, doctors confronted Eric about this again, where he categorically denied injecting himself, stating that neither had anyone else. There is a condition, factitious insulin-induced hypoglycaemia, whereby insulin is injected by either the individual or someone else for the purposes of attention or sympathy (Marks, 1992). It was felt that this could be the case with Eric.

Unfortunately, the blood sample taken from Eric at post mortem for laboratory testing could not be used because the red blood cells had burst (haemolysis), contaminating the sample and making it useless for insulin or C-peptide analysis. A second set of samples were also unfit for testing. This meant that insulin overdose could not be ruled out as this was not tested for. Urine tests taken at the two post mortems were also tested and were found to contain varying amounts of insulin, although the C-peptide content was similar. However, Marks and Richmond (2007) have stated that at this time, there was no knowledge regarding how much insulin is contained in urine during life because this was considered an unreliable measurement. Comparisons were undertaken with the urine of other corpses and, whilst the C-peptide level was similar, Eric's urine sample contained far more insulin than the control specimens.

It was determined that the amount of insulin and C-peptide in the urine was not the same as that in the bloodstream. It was also impossible to determine whether hypoglycaemia had led to Eric's death because this cannot be diagnosed in a cadaver (Marks, 2005). Evidence emerged that Maria had lied about working on the night Eric died and that she had actually been with another man. At the trial, Maria's former husband testified that she had threatened to kill him with an injection of insulin between the toes where the marks would not be found and, as with nurse and possible murderer, Kenneth Barlow, Maria had bragged to nursing colleagues many times that this would be an easy way to kill. This was especially a strong possibility because nurse, Beverly Allitt, had done exactly that only a few years before. On May 22, 1997, Maria was convicted of Eric's murder although no injection marks were identified and despite the patchy evidence.

## AN INSULIN SUICIDE?

In August, 1995, a 34-year old Englishwoman was found close to death by her landlord. He had entered her room after hearing choking sounds, then promptly called an ambulance. By the time it arrived, the woman had stopped breathing and she was dead, certified by her own doctor who was also called. Nothing suspicious was felt to have occurred. However, because the death was unexpected, a post mortem was carried out. The only unusual finding was congestion of the lungs (pulmonary oedema) which was felt to be associated with the death, but not the cause of it (Marks and Richmond, 2007). The woman's landlord, and his partner, reported that the deceased had been an alcoholic. She was also taking prescribed tranquilizers, and was self-medicating with sleeping pills.

It was ascertained that the landlord's partner had Type 1 diabetes and that insulin was kept in the house shared with the deceased. The pathologist conducting the post mortem knew this and had extracted some of the vitreous humour from the woman's eyes, wrongly believed to be a precise indicator of blood glucose level at the time of death (Marks and Richmond, 2007). The level of glucose measured was 0.12mmol/L (2mg/dl). However, blood glucose levels are not the same in death as they are in life, and this was not unusual in someone who had been dead for more than 24 hours (Madea and Rödig, 2006). Because the level of glucose in the vitreous humour of the corpse was so low, administration of insulin was suspected to have contributed towards the woman's death.

A blood sample was sent for C-peptide and insulin analysis, but not for glucose as the blood was obtained after death. The concentration of insulin in the sample was determined at a very high 17 units per litre, with an undetectable C-peptide concentration, meaning that the insulin had been injected (Marks and Richmond, 2007). The woman's body was re-examined but no injection marks were found. However, a number of tissue samples were taken and found to contain small amounts of insulin, whilst one from the area of the right hip was found to contain a large concentration of insulin. The post mortem had confirmed that the woman had been sexually active the night before her death, and her landlord later admitted that this was indeed the case, although he had not forced the woman to do so.

An open verdict was recorded concerning the death, although it was clear that a huge dose of insulin had either caused or contributed to it (Marks and Richmond, 2007). It appeared to be suicide, as the woman would have been aware of being injected if this had been malicious, and she had time to call an ambulance herself before the insulin took effect. However, no injection equipment or insulin were found at the scene, although the woman may have intentionally hidden these, and no suicide note was found, if indeed one was written. Because alcohol had also been ingested, this assisted the insulin in lowering blood glucose levels to a degree that caused unconsciousness and death. Marks and Richmond (2007) have suggested that the woman may have killed herself with insulin after having sex with her landlord and hidden the syringe and insulin vial in order to implicate him in her murder. Unfortunately the question of whether this was a suicide or a murder will never be answered.

## A PERSON WITH DIABETES DIES SUSPICIOUSLY

In Oxfordshire, 68-year old Norman Harvey died on May 3, 1996 in the council flat that he shared with three other people. Norman lived with 36-year old Susan Shickle, her partner Mark and her child, having an on-off relationship with Susan after she was evicted from her own flat. Susan had made a telephone call to inform her son that she had killed Norman and he told his father, who promptly informed the police. Norman's doctor certified the death and found nothing out of the ordinary, but because death was not expected, Norman's body underwent a post mortem examination. Norman had suffered from Type 2 diabetes for 20 years, having treated the condition with twice-daily insulin injections for four years when his glucose-reducing tablets failed to work sufficiently.

Despite insulin resistance, Norman had been admitted to hospital seven times due to severe hypoglycaemia. Because of this, an alternative anti-diabetes drug was prescribed and Norman was advised to stop taking his insulin. At post mortem, recent injection sites were found on one of Norman's legs (Marks and Richmond, 2007). Susan was charged with Norman's murder and a second post mortem was undertaken to collect blood and tissue samples from the injection sites. The blood glucose level was recorded as 1.9mmol/L (34mg/dl) which was normal in a cadaver (Marks, 2006). Vitreous humour glucose was also very low and this, together with the evidence of Susan's confession to her son, led hypoglycaemia to be cited as the cause of death, although this was contested as being due to lung and coronary heart disease seen at post mortem.

Evidence was given by witnesses at the trial to show that Susan had been annoyed with Norman, and had threatened to kill him. Within the next half-an-hour Susan had drawn insulin into a syringe and entered Norman's bedroom with it. Although Norman emerged from his room a couple of times, Susan had urged him back in and, by the next morning, he was dead. Specimens tested from Norman's body showed that he had also ingested sleeping pills and tranquillizers before his death. Blood tests for insulin revealed the presence of 812 units per ml of blood. A further sample tested using radioimmunoassay found 100-500 times the amount of insulin expected in someone who has not recently eaten (Marks and Richmond, 2007). No insulin was found in the tissue samples retrieved at the second post mortem, and only a small amount from the first. This discrepancy cast doubt on the results. However, evidence was given at the trial by someone claiming to have witnessed the injection of insulin by Susan into Norman. On February 25, 1997, Susan was found guilty of murder and was sentenced to life imprisonment (Marks and Richmond, 2007).

## MURDER IN JAPAN

In 1996 a 25-year old man was found dead with vials of insulin and tranquilizer tablets scattered around his body. The evidence suggested that insulin had been injected in a suicide attempt, but a post mortem examination found air bubbles in the man's heart and the blood vessels of his lungs which the victim could not have achieved himself (Marks and Richmond, 2007). The man's partner was a nurse and confessed to killing her boyfriend. Bizarrely she had first given him tranquilizers in a drink, then set up an intravenous drip containing glucose, given him more tranquilizers and a drug to lower blood pressure. Then she had injected 1,200 units of long-acting (rather than fast-acting) insulin.

Because her partner did not die quickly, she injected him with air. The post mortem found that the insulin to C-peptide ration was dispropor-tionate, showing twice as much insulin to C-peptide when the amount after death would usually be around 20 times more insulin to C-peptide (Iwase et al, 2001). The amounts of insulin and C-peptide found would not have led to a conviction on their own, but the confession and evidence of air bubbles discovered at post mortem resulted in a long prison sentence for the murderess. Marks and Richmond have stated that, if the large amount of insulin had been injected into the tissues rather than intravenously, it would not have disappeared from the body so quickly and would have been present at post mortem.

## THE RIGHT CONVICTION?

An English nurse, Deborah Winzar, stood accused of murdering another nurse, her husband, Dominic McCarthy, in 2000. Dominic had tragically become a paraplegic after a motorcycle accident in 1984, before the pair were married. He was awarded compensation and they moved home, where Deborah became a nursing sister and Dominic was employed as a social worker; they had a son. In January 1997 whilst his wife was at work, Dominic was found unconscious at home and died nine days afterwards. His wife was charged with his murder. The case was referred for trial at Crown Court, but not until July 2000, three-and-a half years after Dominic's death.

After Dominic was found on January 31, 1997, he was admitted to hospital in a hypoglycaemic coma, although the cause was undetermined. Dominic had been suffering from a chest condition and it is known that hypoglycaemia can be caused by severe infection (Marks and Teale, 2001). Dominic was also classed as obese, weighing 20 stones (280 pounds) and also, due to his paralysis, had to use a catheter to empty his bladder, leading to numerous bladder infections. Although Dominic felt tired and unwell on January 30, his wife had arranged to go to a party with a female friend and stay overnight at her house (as she was working close by the next day) whilst her husband stayed at home to look after their child, Tony.

Dominic was found the next morning by Tony's teacher because he had not arrived at nursery school. The GP was called and Deborah arrived back after being contacted. She emptied Dominic's catheter bag, which was full. A hypodermic needle was found lying by the bedroom door. As Dominic was struggling to breathe, he was given oxygen by the ambulance crew, another situation (oxygen depletion) that could also have been the cause of his hypoglycaemia (Marks and Richmond, 2007). A blood glucose test revealed that Dominic had severe hypoglycaemia and he was given intravenous glucose and three glucose injections. He was also started on powerful antibiotics. Unusually, he remained in a deep coma, which had lasted for over three hours. A C.T. scan showed that Dominic had swelling of the brain.

Throughout her husband's hospital stay, Deborah was a concerned and caring wife. It was thought that death was due to vomit inhaled during severe hypoglycaemia, although the cause could also have been severe infection, masked in blood samples by the action of strong antibiotics. A blood sample was tested for glucose and found to be 0.7mmol/L (13mg/dl), meaning there was no doubt about the hypoglycaemia, only the cause. There was a large amount of C-peptide in a urine sample which suggested that the insulin present was produced by Dominic himself, although the sample may have been collected after glucose treatment, meaning natural insulin could have been produced in response. When immunoassay test results were received, however, these indicated that the insulin was not naturally produced and it therefore seemed likely that it had been injected. The police became involved and a further test sample threw up different results, showing that the insulin might have have been injected after all.

Despite this, routine tests conducted on Dominic every day indicated that severe infection had been present because of albumin leakage through the capillaries, which does not occur in coma due to insulin overdose (Marks and Richmond, 2007). At post mortem, no abnormalities were found in Dominic's liver, the only organ that can show irrefutably that hypoglycaemia is the cause of death due to certain characteristic changes (Marks, 2005). A total of three post mortem examinations were conducted, with respiratory distress initially cited as the cause of death. It was later thought that Dominic had received a fatal dose of insulin and that his wife was the prime suspect. Deborah Winzar was eventually charged with her husband's murder on January 29, 1998 and was released on bail until her trial which lasted six weeks, finally being sentenced to a minimum of fifteen years imprisonment.

Although no needle marks were found, because Dominic was obese it would have taken at least 1,000 units of injected insulin to kill him (Marks and Richmond, 2007). The evidence that Dominic vomited suggests he did not have hypoglycaemia as the stomach empties quickly in this case to raise blood glucose levels; plasma potassium levels were also normal, contrary to the usual low levels seen in hypoglycaemia; and Dominic had also produced a large quantity of urine which would not occur with severe hypoglycaemia due to the simultaneous release of antidiuretic (water retention) hormone (Marks, 2005). Despite this, and although there was no motive for murder, the fact that Dominic did not recover when glucose was administered suggests that there was too much insulin present, potentially injected insulin. As with all deaths involving hypoglycaemia, the presence of severe infection also contributed towards his death. There is no explanation for Dominic's hypoglycaemia. An appeal against the conviction was launched in 2006 on the grounds that no injection site was located, but this was lost when the judge decided that this was "no basis for declaring the verdict unsafe".

## WERE BOTH ALCOHOL AND INSULIN TO BLAME?

In April, 2000, a middle-aged woman died in Wales. She had an unfortunate history of bad relationships and used large quantities of alcohol as a coping mechanism. After a particularly drunken evening with friends the woman was helped into bed and that was the last time she was seen alive. An ambulance was called but paramedics could not revive her. Although her heart had stopped, the woman was given glucose, adrenaline and an antidote to heroin poisoning in case this was related to her condition;

blood glucose levels were found to be negligible, although it was not known how long she had been dead (Marks and Richmond, 2007).

Evidence revealed that a member of the drinking party had recklessly brought a bottle of insulin along with him and suggested he inject the group to give them a high. This is the case because of the adrenaline that is released during hypoglycaemia (Wilson, 2011). Syringes had been left in the house by a former resident who took drugs, and with both insulin and a means to inject it, the "party" commenced. Several of the friends experienced the symptoms of hypoglycaemia in the hours that followed. A post mortem examination of the dead woman was conducted, identifying alcohol-related changes in the liver; the injection mark was also spotted. The woman's blood insulin level did not correspond to the fact that she had not eaten, confirming what was already known: that insulin was injected.

Although it is not known how much insulin was given, it would not have been enough to kill on its own. Insulin taken with a large amount of alcohol was the deadly combination. Tests confirmed that blood glucose levels were not fatally lowered by alcohol because of the amount of insulin present in the woman's blood. In addition, beta-hydroxide, which appears in the blood when someone dies from alcohol-related hypoglycaemia, was not present (Marks and Richmond, 2007). As a result of his foolish actions, the injector of the insulin was charged with manslaughter and was sentenced to two years imprisonment. He later appealed against his conviction on the grounds that insulin is a natural substance and because the victim had agreed to be injected, but he was unsuccessful (Marks and Richmond, 2007).

## Trust me, I'm a doctor

In a change from the insulin crimes occasionally perpetuated by nurses, Dr Colin Bouwer from New Zealand used insulin to kill his wife in 2001. Colin was a psychiatrist, but had the power to write prescriptions, leaving him free to write one for insulin on behalf of his non-diabetic 47-year old wife, Annette. Bouwer had tried to cover his tracks by contacting a number of hypoglycaemia experts, claiming that a patient of his had died in her sleep after an injection of insulin 7–12 hours before, and asking if this could be cited as the cause of death. Bouwer was charged with this crime and evidence emerged that he had also tried to achieve death by hypoglycaemia over several weeks using glucose-lowering drugs.

However, the defence lawyers felt Annette's hypoglycaemia was due to an undiagnosed and untreated insulin-secreting tumour which had not been apparent at post mortem. They also suggested that Annette may have attempted suicide using medication Dr Bouwer had intended for his own suicide because of his wife's ongoing ill-health. In November 1999 an ambulance had been called after Annette was found deeply unconscious with a blood glucose level of 1.3mmol/L (23mg/dl). She was given glucose orally and glucagon to stimulate glucose release from the liver by injection, increasing her blood glucose to 5.5mmol/L (99mg/dl) when she reached hospital. Later that evening Annette's blood glucose fell to 2.6mmol/L (47mg/dl) and, although conscious, she was given intravenous glucose, raising the level to 14.5mmol/l (261mg/dl). Annette told doctors that she had recently gained weight because she was very hungry, particularly at night. Hypoglycaemia due to alcohol or other medications was ruled out. Her blood glucose level continued to yo-yo between severe hypoglycaemia and 8mmol/L (144mg/dl).

Annette was discharged and advised to eat little and often to avoid hypoglycaemia and was issued with a blood glucose meter so that she could check her levels during the night. Four days later however, Annette was back in hospital suffering similar periodic hypoglycaemic events that were often severely low. This remained the case despite her eating normally whilst a glucose drip remained in place. The symptoms were consistent with an insulinoma, although one could not be found after numerous tests, but these can, very rarely, develop outside the pancreas (Marks and Richmond, 2007). It was suggested that Annette was, for some reason, lying about the results of her own finger-prick blood tests and she was put on a fast with venous blood being taken only if she had a low capillary reading (Marks and Richmond, 2008c).

As a result, Annette's blood glucose levels remained within the normal range and she was discharged on Christmas Eve, 1999 with medication to assist her digestion as a significant portion of her pancreas had been removed for testing. By January 2000, the same thing was happening again and Dr Bouwen collected a venous blood sample from Annette for glucose testing, which measured 1.7mmol/L (31mg/dl), although the sample was blighted by haemolysis. Colin found Annette dead on January 5. She had vomited (implying no hypoglycaemia), although traces of glucose gel were found on her lips. The family doctor certified Annette's death as due to hypoglycaemia and an undetected insulinoma.

Many aspects of Annette's hypoglycaemia were not investigated and the case finally came to trial almost two years after her death. It emerged that Colin had wanted to kill Annette so that he could be with another woman and collect a substantial sum in insurance. The defence put forward the suggestion that Annette had, in fact, suffered from a rare condition (insulin hyperplasia) where the insulin-producing cells of the pancreas are unusually enlarged, giving rise to frequent hypoglycaemia (Marks and Richmond, 2007). However, the evidence of numerous prescriptions for blood glucose lowering substances, traceable back to Dr. Bouwer, was suspicious. Bouwer was known to be a liar and had previously told people that Annette was dying of a terminal condition. He had also telephoned his mother-in-law before Annette's death to say that she was ill and would die before Annette's mother could reach New Zealand to see her daughter. Dr Colin Bouwer was found guilty of his wife's murder and was awarded a mandatory life sentence (Marks and Richmond, 2008c). As so often occurs, the behaviour of the killer, in this case, a telephone call, became evidence of Bouwer's guilt.

## EUTHANASIA OF THE VULNERABLE

In two hospitals in the North of England, a total of four elderly and infirm patients died during 2001–2002 after they were given enough insulin to kill them; and a further 90-year old patient narrowly escaped this fate. The person responsible was a nurse involved in their care, 32-year old Colin Norris. So blasé was Norris about his actions that he actually boasted his prediction of the death of one patient, 86-year old Ethel Hall, who later slipped into a hypoglycaemic coma. He was finally convicted on suspicion of the deaths of Mrs Hall; 80-year old Doris Ludlum; 88-year old Bridget Bourke; and 79-year old Irene Crooks in March 2008 and was given a life sentence (Ford, 2008). Norris was said to have been influenced to kill the frail with insulin by the intriguing trial of nurse, Jessie McTavish.

## A CRIME OF PASSION

In 2002 another nurse received a life-sentence in the USA for the murder of her husband's mistress. Vicki Jensen's husband had left her to co-habit with the other woman and Vicki assumed that doing away with the mistress would bring her husband back. As appears to have happened all too often in these cases, Vicki had previously threatened to murder her husband's ex-wife with insulin. Two years later Vicki was again plotting to murder and involved her young niece and the niece's boyfriend in the crime. When Vicki's husband was known to be safely out of the way at work, the three co-conspirators visited the home he now shared with his mistress and overpowered her whilst the nurse performed an injection of insulin and methamphetamine (a powerful stimulant). Vicki then placed the empty bottle of methamphetamine in her love rival's handbag so it appeared that it belonged to her.

In a twist of fate, evidence given by the niece and her boyfriend told of the mistress's desperation on being injected as she had an allergy to the stimulant. The two assistants later left when the mistress was comatose, leaving Vicki alone. Vicki Jensen escaped the death penalty, receiving a fixed life sentence (Marks and Richmond, 2007). As the victim lay dying, her three-year old daughter was encouraged to watch, and this was cited as the reason why Vicki's appeal for a reduced sentence failed. Her niece's boyfriend received a sentence of 15 years, and her niece a sentence of 12 years. The mistress may have died because of her allergy to methamphetamine alone, had Vicki known about this. The addition of hypoglycaemia, however, ensured she was successful.

**TECHNOLOGY PLAYS ITS PART**

Insulin pump therapy is a device that delivers insulin continuously under the skin in amounts set by the individual and their health professional. In 2004, Butch et al highlighted the use of insulin pump technology to deliver lethal doses of the drugs Etomidate and Atracurium into two individuals, causing their deaths. Etomidate is a short-acting intravenous anaesthetic used to render a patient anaesthetised or sedated for procedures such as relocating dislocated joints. The drug has been associated with increased mortality due to suppression of the adrenal system (Morris and McAllister, 2005). Atracurium besylate is a skeletal muscle relaxant used during surgical procedures and mechanical ventilation (Hughes, 1986). Administered continuously by insulin pump technology, the effects of both drugs were lethal, added to the fact that the individuals were also not receiving what they though was their insulin.

**INSULIN MURDER OR UNDERLYING CONDITION?**

In 2011, a number of patients in the care of 27-year old nurse, Rebecca Leighton, were found to have unexpectedly low blood glucose levels in Steeping Hill Hospital, Greater Manchester. An investigation found intravenous saline drip bags had been contaminated with insulin, meaning the victims were not specifically chosen; it was the luck of the draw. Three patients had died but also suffered from underlying medical conditions making death more likely: 83-year-old Alfred Derek Weaver; 71-year old Arnold Lancaster; and 44-year old Tracey Arden. A further two deaths were subsequently linked to the murder investigation. It was discovered that very early on July 22, a further 14 saline bags were found to have been injected with insulin, suggesting that an unknown number of patients may have died as a result of the contamination.

Leighton was charged with three counts of criminal damage and intent to endanger life; three counts of criminal damage being reckless as to whether life was being endangered; and one charge of theft (Carter, 2012). She was remanded in custody but the charges were later dropped in September as it was felt no longer appropriate to continue the case due to insufficient evidence. On December 2, it emerged that Leighton had been dismissed from her nursing position having been on suspension for five months. Police were now investigating a total of 19 possible deaths from insulin-contaminated saline and by July 2012, 22 cases had been revealed with a total of eight deaths, all vulnerable on the acute care wards. Leighton spent six weeks in prison but was cleared of the murder charges and released, but she did admit to stealing drugs and medicines from the hospital. The nurse who had been contaminating the saline bags with insulin was 48-year old Victorino Chua, who was held on suspicion of three counts of murder and 18 counts of grievous bodily harm. He had also tampered with patients' medical records so that they received more medication than was necessary. His bail was extended a total of five times until November 2013 (BBC, 2013).On March 28, 2014, Chua was re-arrested and charged with three counts of murder and 31 other offences.

# CHAPTER SIX

# THE HIGHS AND LOWS OF INSULIN MISUSE IN FICTION

The dramatic effect of insulin overdose is very appealing to fiction writers in books, film and television. Unfortunately the depictions of hypoglycaemia, hyperglycaemia, or even diabetes as a condition, are frequently unrealistic and there is little space within the plot for explanation. This can give the impression that those who take insulin are careless with their treatment and that potential murderers have easy access to the individual's insulin supply and are proficient in knowing how to inject it and how much would kill. Detective fiction and crime drama plots also exploit the action of insulin in lowering blood glucose levels as a potential murder weapon that will be very difficult for the police and medical science to detect.

As seen with true-life murder cases involving insulin, it is practically impossible for insulin to kill a person without other factors contributing towards death, such as an underlying medical condition, old age, alcohol and drug consumption, or insulin overdose in addition to situations such as drowning. The 1970s television crime drama, *A Man Called Ironside*, stated in one episode that insulin was the perfect way to kill someone because as a murder weapon, it was untraceable. In 1974 this belief led nurse, Jessie McTavish, otherwise known as "The Angel of Death", to kill 80-year old Elizabeth Lyon with insulin and to inject three other patients because she thought her crimes could never be detected. McTavish actually admitted that she had got the idea of an insulin murder from the television show and, as a consequence of this case, Nurse Colin Norris killed a total of four patients with insulin in 2001–2002 in the North of England. Norris claimed that his actions were driven by the use of insulin in the McTavish case. These are just two incidences of the dangers of truth mimicking fiction.

Television drama shows periodically run a story line about someone with Type 1 diabetes where there is hypoglycaemia involved, and great emphasis is placed on whether the person will be found in time to save them; it is edge of the seat viewing. An episode of the English detective drama, *A Tough of Frost*, with actor David Jason playing the lead character, showed a plot where a woman with Type 1 diabetes was kidnapped one morning. She had injected herself with her dose of insulin but not actually eaten anything, then drove off in her car before being abducted. This of course is completely at odds with what any sensible person with Type 1 diabetes would do in case their blood glucose level became low when driving.

The kidnapper took his victim to a disused warehouse and left her there without any means of communicating with the outside world and, of course, with no food or insulin for almost three days. In a race against time, Detective Inspector Frost tracked down where the woman was being held and, as would be expected after this length of time without insulin, the woman was panting when found. This would seem due to high blood glucose levels and ketoacidosis, but much was made of low blood glucose levels, although entirely the wrong symptoms were depicted. A policeman handed the woman a chocolate bar and she quickly ate it, nodding that she had made a very quick recovery, although perhaps this was just hunger. This is, of course, a completely unrealistic portrayal of what would happen to someone diabetes-wise if these frightening circumstances actually arose.

Similarly in a BBC production of the English daytime show, *Doctors,* an elderly woman with Type 1 diabetes and arthritis decided to kill herself using her medication. Although having other medical conditions and being elderly would hasten a death from insulin, the portrayal was typically difficult to believe. In an earlier episode of the same show, a young man with Type 1 diabetes was told by his doctor about insulin pump therapy, a subcutaneous method of delivering measured dosages of insulin to meet the individual's needs to enable tighter control of blood glucose levels, because it was felt this would enable him to manage his condition far better. Factually however, the information portrayed was wrong and the individual was an unlikely candidate for this treatment as he was not prepared to monitor his blood glucose levels regularly and act upon the results. Diabetes appears numerous times in fiction, with almost forty films alone depicting a character with diabetes (Ferguson, 2010). The following examples of diabetes in fiction are chosen because they demonstrate the perpetuation of certain beliefs about the condition, about how a murder could go undetected with insulin (although this is false), or they show the realities of life for the sufferer.

## THE CASE OF THE MISSING WILL (1925)

Agatha Christie trained as a pharmacy dispenser before becoming possibly the best writer of crime fiction that there has ever been. With her pharmaceutical knowledge Christie was well aware of substances which could be used to murder without suspicion and always used this expert knowledge in her stories and books. This is especially true at the time of her first writing about an insulin murder in the mid-1920s, only four years after the discovery of the hormone by Banting and Best in 1921. Although Christie usually packed her tales with murder, in this short story, which was later adapted for television in 1993, only one person dies, and it is due in part to insulin. For the purposes of context, the plot is as follows.

Andrew Marsh, a very wealthy copper seam owner, gathers his family and friends together as the New Year chimes in on January 1, 1926. He, for some reason, announces the contents of his will: three-quarters of Marsh's money is left to his good friend and physician Dr Pritchard and his Elinfort Medical Foundation. One thousand pounds is left to two young boys, Peter Baker and Robert Siddaway, who are the sons of family friends and will each receive their inheritance when they are 18. One person who is only left a small trust fund is Violet Wilson, the child of Marsh's business partner and a ward of Andrew Marsh following the death of her father. This story is set in the times when women were fighting for equal rights with men and it is assumed that, because Violet is a woman, she will marry and her husband will provide for her.

Ten years have passed and all the children have grown up. In 1936, Peter Baker is now in the army and Robert Siddaway and Violet Wilson are now students at Cambridge University. The Cambridge Union is a chauvinist place at this time; women cannot be accorded equal status to men. Because this was the case, women were not granted the honour of having a graduation ceremony once they had completed their university degrees. Women were also not allowed to apply for a bank loan in their own name without a husband or father to agree to be guarantor. Violet is portrayed as a staunch feminist campaigner who produces a magazine, *New Prospects*. Her efforts, entirely without male assistance, are supported by college principal, Miss Phillyda Campion as Violet is unable to borrow the money she needs to produce the magazine independently and run her own publishing enterprise.

Andrew Marsh, often breathless due to a serious heart condition, decides to revise his former will, leaving everything to Violet because of her academic achievements at Cambridge University. All of the former guests and beneficiaries at the previous revelation of the contents of Marsh's will are present in the house. Dr Pritchard is called when Marsh has even more difficulty than usual in breathing and leaves his medical bag unattended in the hallway whilst examining his patient. Andrew Marsh is told that his life is drawing to a close. The great detective, Hercule Poirot, is also staying with Marsh, who invites his old friend to be an executor to his new will, telling Poirot of his intention to leave everything to Violet. Later that night at half-past midnight, Marsh receives a mysterious telephone call asking him to meet someone at the folly in the extensive grounds of his country house. Although he tries to bargain for a better time, and although he continues to feel unwell, Marsh forces himself to go outside and meet this person, but is found dead the next morning. Dr Pritchard states that there is no need for a post mortem as he had recently seen Marsh for his heart complaint. Poirot carries out a thorough inspection of the area around the body but finds nothing unusual. There are, as with all of Christie's plots, many suspects in Poirot's eyes, although Marsh's doctor is in no doubt that Marsh's passing is due to natural causes and cites heart failure on the death certificate. When the family gather to hear the reading of the original will which is the only such document because the new one was never written, it appears to be missing, meaning that Marsh died intestate. Poirot states that Andrew Marsh had changed his will and, with his usual tenacity, scours the folly where his friend died once more. He manages to find an empty medical vial with numbers embossed on the glass. Poirot then becomes convinced that his friend was murdered.

After the numbers of the medical vial are traced by the police, it transpires that the bottle had contained insulin, the kind of sample once distributed to doctors. However, keeping insulin, (which is a protein) inside a medical bag for weeks, if not months on end, would render its action diminished if it became warm. For this reason it is advisable to store insulin in a fridge, but the domestic fridge did not become popular until the turn of the century once there was a reliable electricity supply. In a later Agatha Christie story from 1936, fridges were still not in widespread use in the home and were seen as something of a novelty.

In *The Case of the Missing Will,* Dr Pritchard tells Poirot that Andrew Marsh had a son, and that he, the doctor, did not kill him for the money Marsh was leaving to his Medical Foundation. Poirot concludes that Dr. Pritchard could not be the murderer as he was the major beneficiary of the will. He decides that if he finds out who is Marsh's son, he will find the murderer. After asking many questions the plot unravels. Poirot discovers that Peter Baker is not Andrew Marsh's son, as suspected, because he was conceived whilst Marsh was away. He finds that Marsh did have a son with Sarah Siddaway, a children's nurse hired to look after Violet when she was younger, meaning that Robert Siddaway would have inherited Marsh's fortune as his heir.

Miss Campion, principal of the ladies' college attended by Violet Wilson at Cambridge University, is pushed down an escalator and breaks her leg. Poirot discovers that Phyllida Campion also had a child out of wedlock with Marsh and that Violet Wilson is Marsh's daughter. Former children's nurse, Sarah Siddaway, who was still working for Andrew Marsh, had tried to kill Miss Campion so that she would not tell anyone that Violet was due to inherit her father's fortune. When the doctor had been called to see Marsh, Sarah Siddaway had rifled through his unattended medical bag, taking a glass and stainless steel syringe and the bottle of insulin.

The former nurse had telephoned and arranged to meet Marsh. She had then somehow managed to inject him with what was described as "a massive and fatal dose" of insulin because she knew the power of the drug. With Marsh's weak heart, although the syringe was only about one-third full, and Marsh was injected through a thick tweed jacket and his other clothes, this was enough to kill. Because of Sarah Siddaway's actions, her son Robert did not inherit Marsh's fortune. All ends happily though with Violet Wilson graduating from Cambridge University in a special ceremony just for women, then using her large inheritance to fund the regular publication of *New Prospects,* setting herself up as the Chairwoman of her own publishing company.

## MURDER IS EASY (1939)

This book and later television adaptation in 2008 is again by Agatha Christie and is set during the Second World War when regular insulin supplies were sometimes hard to come by for patients, although the hospitals practising insulin coma therapy at this time did not have the same problem. To put this shortage for people with Type 1 diabetes into context, when The Phillipines was invaded by Japan at the beginning of the Second World War, insulin had to be obtained by pulverising pig pancreases to form an injectable substance that was at least better than nothing, although it was difficult to gauge correct dosages. Whilst the situation was not quite so dire in rural England, in Christie's book, *Murder is Easy,* a total of seven people are killed to cover up a family secret, one of these murders being achieved using insulin as a contributing factor.

To put this fictional death by hypoglycaemia into context, the background plot is as follows. In the picturesque village of Wychwood, the community is very close-knit and everyone seems aware of the other villager's business. When a young man with learning difficulties, Leonard Waynflete, is drowned in a fast-flowing river, it is assumed that he slipped to his death on the rocks. Twenty-two years later, an attractive girl arrives in the village under the pretence of touring local churches on a brass-rubbing holiday. When she begins to ask personal questions about several of the local women, suspicions are raised and the person most rattled is Honoria Waynflete, sister of the drowned Leonard. A spate of seemingly unrelated deaths soon follow.

First to die is the resident wise woman, Florrie Gibbs, who is renowned for her knowledge of herbs and natural medications to "help people out". Despite her knowledge, Florrie dies after eating a stew containing mushrooms which she has picked from the forest. This unexpected death is naturally attributed to a terrible accident. Local vicar, the Reverend Minchin, is a keen bee-keeper, but he is unfortunately gassed when wearing his protective bee-keeper's mask. Again, this tragedy and loss of the well-loved, kind and long-serving Reverend within the village is put down to pure accident.

The village gossip, Lavinia Pinkerton, meets Miss Jane Marple on a train and tells her all about the vicar's death, adding that she is sure it was not an accident. This rouses Marple's curiosity for a mystery and she visits the village to observe the goings on at first hand. Lavinia later visits Honoria Waynflete for afternoon tea and speculates wildly about the two recent deaths in the village, again stating that she feels this is very suspicious and that a visit to the police is definitely called for. Climbing onto a crowded escalator after getting off a train, Lavinia is viciously pushed from behind and she falls to her death. Honoria's cat has been suffering from an infected ear and the next unfortunate individual to die in the village is the local physician, Doctor Humbleby. Whilst visiting Honoria, he badly cuts his finger as some crockery is smashed, and she applies a dressing which is not as sterile as it could have been, causing the poor man to develop blood poisoning.

As if four unfortunate deaths in a close community were not enough, a fifth occurs when Amy Gibbs, grand-daughter of wise woman Florrie and maid to Honoria Waynflete, becomes ill. She develops a persistent cough which the killer uses as an ideal opportunity to remove another person from the village. Amy takes to swallowing cough medicine in large doses in an effort to shift the irritation, and also happens to have a hat that she wishes to dye to change its colour. Her employer, Honoria, kindly offers her some red hat dye to do the job, but sadly, the dye is contained in a bottle exactly the same shape and size as the cough medicine. With inevitably and dramatic consequences, Amy drinks from the wrong bottle in the middle of the night and is found dead the next morning with red dye spewing from her mouth. Yet again, this is felt to be nothing more than a terrible accident.

The sixth and final unfortunate village member to be dispatched is Lydia Horton, the local councillor's wife and Type 1 diabetes sufferer. In line with other insulin murders in fiction, the method and dosage are questionable, as are the circumstances, although Marks and Richmond (2007) in their excellent book, *Insulin Murders: True Life Cases,* do state that most insulin murders occur because of a combination of factors, which is the case with Lydia Horton. Having injected herself from a huge 1000 unit bottle of insulin and a stainless steel and glass syringe with 60 units of insulin with no food consumed, she climbs into a hot bath after drinking a quantity of whisky, both factors (alcohol and hot baths) known to rapidly reduce blood glucose levels and accelerate the action of insulin. Marks and Richmond (2007) have stated that a reduction in blood glucose level can be seen after drinking only six units (150ml/50g) of whisky.

Having already successfully acted to personally induce a level of hypoglycaemia, Lydia is unfortunate enough to become the sixth victim of the killer who injects a total of 300 units of insulin into Lydia's big toe. It is very difficult to believe that a whole 300 units of insulin could be forced under the skin of the big toe, there being little subcutaneous fat in this area of hard tissue. However, the police report stated that Lydia died after drinking alcohol and being injected with 300 units of insulin. It is not explained how this was calculated from a 1,000 unit bottle, in addition to the 60 units that Lydia injected herself.

There was no depiction of any symptoms of hypoglycaemia before her death, this being left to the imagination after leaving the sinister suggestion that insulin was the dangerous substance that had lead to Lydia clearly taking her own life. As mentioned earlier, Marks and Richmond (2007) have stated that it would take up to 1,000 units of insulin to kill someone, depending on their size and insulin sensitivity. In the case of a real-life insulin murder, one wonders whether Maria Whiston was influenced by Agatha Christie when she injected her husband, Eric, between the toes with insulin in 1994 because she thought this was an area of the body where an injection could not be traced.

It is revealed that there had been a total of seven unexpected deaths in this quiet little English village; Miss Marple puts the pieces together and discovers that the murderess was Honoria Waynflete. When challenged,

Honoria confesses, her justification being that after becoming pregnant by her brother, whom she pushed to his death into the fast-flowing river, the result of the union was a daughter. The brass-rubbing enthusiast was in actual fact Honoria's offspring, Bridget Conway, seeking her mother after 22 years. Honoria was still so shamed by having had a child with her brother that she had attempted to remove everyone in the village who knew, or might have known, her dreadful secret so that Bridget did not discover the truth.

Florrie Gibbs had been murdered after supplying Honoria with a tincture of mugwort in order to bring about abortion. However, Honoria had decided not to take the substance and had distracted Florrie by ringing the doorbell so she could slip the poisonous mushrooms into Florrie's stew because she knew Honoria had been pregnant by her brother. The Reverend Minchin was also removed because Honoria had confessed her sin to him and, although he had sworn to keep her secret, she could not take that risk when Bridget Conway turned up asking awkward questions. Lavinia Pinkerton was a victim of her own nosiness by being so interested in what she considered to be the two suspicious deaths in the village. These absolutely had to be reported to the police, and she was the woman to do it. Honoria had been responsible for pushing Lavinia down the escalator at the train station which, unlike a similar escalator accident in *The Case of The Missing Will* (1925), ended in the death of the victim rather than a broken leg.

Dr Humbleby, although bound by his Hippocratic doctor's oath not to disclose any information about a patient, or the circumstances of a pregnancy, was killed by Honoria just in case he was tempted to share her secret. The fortunate occurrence of her cat's infected ear proved ideal as a source of contaminated material to place on a dressing to put onto the wound on Dr Humbleby's finger. Honoria had deliberately nicked it with a piece of sharp crockery as they both bent to pick up the scattered shards. This resulted in septicaemia and the doctor duly died from his blood poisoning. Honoria's maid, Amy Gibbs, was pregnant when she died. She had visited her grandmother, Florrie, for the same "help" with getting rid of the baby as Honoria had done all those years before. Amy's employer was terrified that Florrie had told Amy that Honoria had been in the same predicament. Although a tenuous link, poor Amy also had to die, being poisoned by the oxalic acid in the red hat dye consumed instead of cough mixture. The final victim, Lydia Horton, died because she happened to be a similar age to Honoria and Bridget Conway felt that Lydia could be her mother. Honoria knew that Bridget would not stop digging until she uncovered the truth about who her mother was, and again, couldn't take the risk of her finding out the truth, although, of course, it all came out in the end, after seven senseless murders.

Agatha Christie had enough knowledge of the power of insulin, even in 1925 (*The Case of the Missing Will*) and 1936 (*Murder is Easy*) to portray her insulin-related murder victims as also having a secondary reason why death had occurred, making this more feasible. In the former, Andrew Marsh had a chronic heart condition making him vulnerable to the insulin he was given. In the latter, Lydia Horton has been drinking heavily before she was injected with the insulin in addition to her own self-administered dosage, meaning the two worked in a deadly alliance to fatally lower her blood glucose levels in a way that would have been survived without alcohol (Marks and Medd, 1964).

## STEEL MAGNOLIAS (1989)

This comedy-drama film revolves around a home-based beauty salon run by Truvy Jones (played by Dolly Parton). Annelle Dupuy (played by Daryl Hannah) is hired to work in the salon, and Truvy's friend, M'Lynn Eatenton (played by Sally Field), and her daughter Shelby (played by Julia Roberts) visit the salon when Shelby is preparing for her wedding. No doubt due to the excitement of the forthcoming event, Shelby experiences moderately severe hypoglycaemia, which is well-acted, whilst having her hair done. She remains conscious and quickly feels well again after drinking fruit juice administered by her mother. As it is later revealed that

Shelby's Type 1 diabetes is not well-controlled it may also be assumed that her hypoglycaemic awareness was impaired due to nerve damage and so Shelby did not realise she was becoming low. This demonstrates to viewers the difficulties of managing the condition, although the problem of absent warning signs of hypoglycaemia are probably not obvious to someone who has never experienced this. It may also be the case that the bride-to-be is too caught up in thoughts of her wedding to be thinking about her diabetes.

Several months after her wedding, Shelby tells her family that she is pregnant, but for her mother, this is not good news because she worries about the effect this will have on Shelby's body. Keeping blood glucose levels stable throughout the nine months of pregnancy with hormonal variations is often very difficult, meaning that if the mother's blood glucose levels are high, the baby grows to a larger size (possibly in the region of one stone or 14 pounds in weight). The baby also produces more waste products because the glucose passing from mother to baby is higher than normal. In *Steel Magnolias*, M'Lynn tells the salon that Shelby had been advised by her diabetes consultant not to have children because of pre-existing kidney disease, a complication of her diabetes caused by continual hyperglycaemia. The salon ponder the fact that Shelby could die because of her pregnancy, but Truvy, ever optimistic, focuses on the happiness of a new baby.

Whilst Shelby survives being pregnant, several months after having given birth to her baby son her kidneys fail and she starts dialysis treatment. Shelby is remarkably upbeat about this and looks very well, hiding the bruises on her arms where the needles are inserted to filter her blood. Whether this is a front because she does not want to talk about her condition; because she is in denial about the seriousness of her diabetes with the evidence that her kidneys have failed; because she does not want others to worry about her, upsetting her mother; or whether she just copes with her situation remarkably well is left to the viewer to determine.

M'Lynn donates one of her kidneys to Shelby and the transplant takes places the day after her son turns one. The transplant has the desired effect and Shelby commences a new lease of life, content with her husband and child. However, there is not a happy ending when, months later, she lifts up her son to hug him and experiences extreme pain. Shelby is later found unconscious by her husband with the telephone grasped in her hand. Sadly, Shelby is in a coma because the new kidney has been rejected and Shelby's family face the agonising decision about removing her life support.

This film is extremely realistic in portraying the issues and consequences related to having chronic complications of diabetes, a subject that is usually left unexplored in fiction. Diabetes is now the leading cause of End Stage Renal Disease (ESRD) in the Western countries and occurs in 25–40 percent of people with Type 1 or Type 2 diabetes (MacIssac and Watts, 2005). After the funeral in *Steel Magnolias*, M'Lynn is devastated and tells the salon girls that Shelby's son will never know what his mother went through to have him. M'Lynn, who had undergone serious surgery to donate one of her kidneys and was still recovering, begins to accept her daughter's death, focussing on her young grandson. Salon worker, Annelle, now married and pregnant herself, asks M'Lynn if she can name her baby after Shelby and, when it is born, the circle of life begins again.

## CHOCOLAT (2000)

This film is a romance based on the novel by Joanne Harris. In a small French village in 1959, Vianne Rocher (played by Juliette Bonoche) and her young daughter Anouk arrive to set up a chocolate shop, just as the 40 days of Lent are due to be observed by the locals. Vianne, who is young and beautiful, has a spectacular talent for making the most delicious chocolate items and she is not at all religious, making her highly unpopular in the village. In addition, when news gets out that Anouk is illegitimate and there is no father-figure on the scene, this does not help Vianne's acceptance in the community. Although it appears that she is receiving disapproving looks and comments from almost everyone around her, Vianne stays remarkably cheerful and her winning personality shines through throughout her long ordeal of trying to be accepted.

Despite her initial effort to gain popularity, the local mayor declares that Vianne is an evil temptress for producing chocolate when the local residents are trying to abstain. Vianne's landlady, Armande (played by Judi Dench) soon discovers how irresistible Vianne's hot chocolate with a sprinkling of chilli is. She tells Vianne that she is not able to see her grandson, Luc, because her own daughter, Caroline, forbids it, saying that Armande is a very bad influence. Vianne steps in to rectify this, unaware of why the problem exists, and she arranges for Luc to see his grandmother at the chocolate shop. When Armande is sitting on a stool in the shop, her daughter marches in to confront her about seeing Luc, and she says how Armande is being negligent as she has Type 1 diabetes and has been told she could be blind within a year, emphasising that she should be in a care home. Caroline snatches at Armande's skirt, but the old woman lifts it herself to reveal several terrible bruises on her legs as a result of her insulin injections, although this does not usually occur unless a blood vessel is punctured.

Armande continues to eat chocolates and drink hot chocolate at the shop because she feels she may as well enjoy life while she can, although seemingly this is a decision to spite her daughter because she has been labelled a bad influence on Luc. Vianne is understanding and offers to throw Armande a party for her 70th birthday, an event Caroline is not invited to. As the long weeks of Lent slip by, the villagers are increasingly tempted by Vianne's chocolates, and they become a secret pleasure for several of the locals. Only the mayor remains strong in his resolution to fast for the entire period of Lent. As the visits to Vianne's shop increase, Luc becomes very close to Armande, but when Caroline discovers that Luc is not in his bed on the night of the party, she rushes round to her mother's house, finding the remains of the get-together.

Vianne becomes friendly with Roux (played by Johnny Depp), one of a band of gypsies who arrive in the village and who are equally unwelcome. When the gypsies hold a party on Roux's boat, an extension of that held for Armande's birthday, Vianne, Anouk, Luc and Armande are present and grandmother and grandson enjoy themselves dancing together. Finding Armande's house empty, Caroline heads for the harbour where she sees there is much jollity and that everyone is enjoying the get-together, including Luc and Armande. Caroline turns away in disgust. Armande tells Luc she is tired and he says he will come with her to do the washing-up from the birthday meal.

As the boy clears the dishes, his grandmother settles in her favourite chair and appears to fall asleep. When Luc comes to tell her he has finished, he finds Armande dead due to her poorly-controlled diabetes. Luc, having only recently got to know his grandmother, finds her death is a terrible blow. At Armande's funeral the priest announces that the congregation must hope that she showed some penitence in her final moments for giving in to the temptations that aggravated her illness and caused her death. The gypsy camp moves on and, still unable to gain any ground with the harsh mayor of the village, Vianne decides to cut her losses and move away.

That night, the mayor breaks into the chocolate shop with the intention of destroying all of the stock so that the villagers have nothing tempting to buy. He inadvertently gets a taste of chocolate crumbs as they land on his lips in his frenzied destruction of the displays. The mayor then gorges on the broken pieces until he finally falls asleep in the window display where Vianne finds him early the next morning. Chocolate contains theobromine which can be toxic. This is poisonous when 300mg of theobromine is consumed per kilogram of bodyweight, but the mayor regains consciousness, although worse for wear. Vianne promises not to breathe a word of his weakness and, with this shared secret and the Mayor's new respect for her confectionary, Vianne and her daughter decide to stay in the village they can now call home.

## MEMENTO (2000)

This is a strange but compelling film about a man, Leonard Shelby (played by Guy Pearce) who completely loses his ability to form short-term memories (retrograde amnesia) after a blow to the head during a break-in and attack in which he thinks his wife was killed. He attempts to piece together all he can find out, although he does not know who he can trust because he feels that people exploit his memory loss to their own ends, for example, paying more than once for the motel room he is staying in. In order to have a permanent record of all the relevant clues he hopes will lead to his wife's killer, he has facts tattooed on his body and takes Polaroid photographs of people and places, writing himself notes such as "Do not trust him".

Before his accident he was an insurance claims investigator and was asked to look into the case of a man with amnesia, Sammy Jankis, whose wife had Type 1 diabetes. The couple were making an insurance claim after Sammy lost his short-term memory and could no longer work. Sammy used to carry out his wife's insulin injections before his memory loss, although she was perfectly capable of doing this herself. Because of this, Shelby had judged their insurance claim invalid as he felt that Sammy should have been able to re-learn tasks by repetition and therefore conditioning because his amnesia was psychological and not physical. Sammy failed to re-learn any tasks and gradually his health worsened, although the health insurance decision held firm. Desperate for money, Sammy's wife begged Shelby (before his accident) to reconsider his decision because it was obvious that Sammy could not learn and retain certain information.

As Leonard Shelby searches for his wife's killer, often going over old ground because he cannot remember the facts, a policeman (John Edward Gammell) helps him in his search. Shelby does not trust him, but tries to do what he can under the circumstances to trace the killer. The case of Sammy Jankis and his wife keeps reappearing throughout the film and, because the case affected Shelby so much, he has had the man's name tattooed on his wrist. In a desperate attempt to make Sammy learn by repetition, his wife tells him it is time for her insulin, although this is strange at 3:20 in the afternoon, unless Sammy's wife took multiple daily injections. Sammy dutifully draws up 17 units from a bottle marked simply "insulin for injection" and his wife rolls up her sleeve so he can inject it, presumably intravenously as she turns her arm to reveal the underside and crook of the elbow.

As a test of memory, Sammy's wife hopes he will remember giving her insulin as he seems to remember how to draw it up and what dosage his wife needs. Twenty minutes later, Sammy's wife says again that it is time for her insulin and Sammy again draws up 17 units of insulin which he injects subcutaneously this time into his wife's abdomen. Twenty minutes later still, the same procedure is repeated and the injection is given into his wife's thigh. Very sadly this exercise to make Sammy realise that his wife had already had her insulin fails. Perhaps Sammy's wife was just tired of getting nowhere with the insurance claim, having no money, and having to look after a husband who now needed her as a full-time carer.

With no sign or symptoms of hypoglycaemia whatsoever after forty minutes since the first injection, and following a total of 51 units of insulin, Sammy's wife rests her head back as she sits of the settee and promptly dies. As seen previously, 51 units of insulin would not be enough to kill on its own, making this film unrealistic in this respect. Sammy is clearly not faking his amnesia as he does not rush to get his wife glucose or phone an ambulance, unless he actually wished to kill his wife and was putting on a very good act. Instead, he sits and stares into space.

As the film draws to a close it is revealed that the police have been using Shelby to hunt down and kill people they would like removed by suggesting, through Gammell, that each target was the person responsible for his wife's death. As vague memories are gradually pieced together, Shelby recalls that he received his head injury when his wife was attacked by an intruder in their bathroom and that his wife did not die in the attack. The twist in the tale is that it was actually Leonard Shelby's wife who had Type 1 diabetes and not Sammy's. With horror, Shelby realises that he was the one who killed his own wife with repeated injections of insulin after she survived the attack by the intruder and that she was the one trying to help Shelby regain his memories by repetitive learning.

## PANIC ROOM (2002)

This film is a thriller starring Jodie Foster as the mother of an 11-year old daughter with Type 1 diabetes. Meg Altman (played by Foster) is newly divorced and wishes to make a fresh start with her daughter Sarah (played by Kristen Stewart) as they move home and relocate to New York. A previous owner of their new property thoughtfully installed a secret reinforced concrete and steel room with surveillance cameras, an intercom system, and a separate telephone line where the occupants could hide in the event that anyone broke into the house. Unfortunately for Meg and Sarah, as they settle into their new home that first evening, they are disturbed by the former owner's grandson, Junior; an employee of the company who installed the security system (Burham); and Raoul, a gunman employed for the job by Junior. The break-in has nothing to do with Meg and her daughter, in fact the trio thought she was not moving in until a later date, giving question to the need for a gunman. The reason for this home invasion is because Junior knows that millions of dollars in bearer bonds are still in the safe and the intruders intend to find them, although why these were not removed when the previous occupant left is not explained. Despite the unexpected find of Altman and her daughter, Junior convinces Burham that they should continue with their plan to seize the bonds whilst the new occupants are sleeping. Meg wakes in the night and sees the three robbers as they enter the house. She wakes Sarah and they rush to the panic room, not realising this is also the intended destination of the intruders.

The pair cannot telephone for help from the separate phone in the room because Junior and his cronies have cut the line. As Meg and Sarah huddle frightened in what is supposed to be a safe haven, the robbers try and fill the small room with propane gas so that the occupants cannot breathe and they can then gain entry. Meg tries to switch off the air vents to the room as Raoul increases the amount of gas seeping in, but this proves unsuccessful. Meg's next plan is to throw a fire blanket over herself and her daughter and ignite the gas inside the room, which causes an explosion to backfire into the room containing the intruders, starting a fire and injuring Junior. After failing to alert the attention of her neighbour by signalling, Meg succeeds in tapping into the main telephone line and phoning her ex-husband (rather than the police) before she is cut off. When Junior is about to give up on the idea of stealing the bearer bonds, Raoul shoots him and urges him to continue. The ex-husband arrives, is taken hostage and is brutally attacked.

To add to the drama, Sarah has a reasonably well-acted severe hypo-glycaemic episode and, of course, there is no form of glucose available in the panic room. Sarah wears a glucose-monitoring watch in the film, which draws attention to the fact that people with Type 1 diabetes must actively self-manage the condition. Fergusson (2010) has suggested that the act of cinemagoers watching the action of diabetes self-care in the film is an allegory of the process of control that diabetes has over the individual and that the individual must have over their diabetes. Meg, no doubt desperate to help her daughter's situation, comes out of the room where she sees her unexpectedly unconscious ex-husband, allowing Burham to enter the room to locate the bearer bonds. He gets more than he bargains for however when he discovers that Sarah is in a state of severe hypoglycaemia, although he doesn't know that is the reason for her state.

In the meantime, Meg gets a glucagon injection kit from the fridge (although her daughter is still conscious and could have eaten glucose tablets, something sweet, or had a sweet drink), and is then intercepted by Raoul who loses his gun in the struggle with her and is somehow thrown into the small room with Burham and Sarah. Meg, in an almighty leap of faith, throws the glucagon kit in after him as Burham locks the door. Over the intercom system Meg asks Burham to give her daughter the glucagon and Sarah, still conscious, rather unbelievably instructs him on how to do it.

As the person with Type 1 diabetes is usually unconscious when glucagon is administered by another person, they are unaware of what needs to be done to prepare it for injection. Whilst the viewer does not see this, this is quite a tricky procedure, especially if the person injecting it has not done this before and in a situation where the unconscious diabetic person is writhing around, twitching and possibly fitting. Any person who has experienced severe hypoglycaemia will know how difficult it is to explain anything, or even speak coherently, as the brain struggles to work in the extreme lack of glucose.

Preparing glucagon for injection requires the glucagon powder to be drawn up from one small bottle, then saline is added from another small bottle to form a solution to be drawn up and injected subcutaneously, although it is also injected intravenously in hospital emergency situations so that it acts even more quickly. If Sarah was this coherent and glucagon was the only available source of glucose, she could have injected herself with it rather than to ask and trust an unknown intruder with no experience. Presumably Meg could also have bargained with the robbers that they could have the bonds, no questions asked, if she could come in and give Sarah the glucagon, but this clearly would have been less dramatic.

Burham gives Sarah the injection, turning him from the predator into the protector, confessing to the girl that his part in the robbery was driven by his desire to be a better provider for his own son. Sarah fortunately recovers with none of the usual post-severe hypoglycaemia headache, counter-regulatory hyperglycaemia, or feeling unwell for a period of several hours afterwards. The police arrive following an earlier call made by Meg's ex-husband and Raoul reacts to this new problem by threatening the kill Sarah. With this in mind, Meg decides to tell the officers that everything is fine and they leave. Burham finally takes the bearer bonds and the robbers take Sarah hostage. Meg attacks Raoul with a sledgehammer as Burham flees with the prize, and Meg is attacked by Raoul in return.

Sarah is obviously distressed and screams out; one would expect her blood glucose levels to be quite high now after the glucagon, hypoglycaemic counter-regulation, and all the stress of the evening. Burham shows that he has a conscience when he comes back to help, shooting Raoul. Burham then makes his escape with the bearer bonds once again. Nothing more is seen of Junior, whose idea the robbery had been in the first place. The police return on cue shortly afterwards because they decide Meg's earlier actions were rather suspicious, given that there were reports of a robbery occurring. The officers manage to capture Burham in the process of leaving the house and he finally gives in, throwing the precious bearer bonds into the air where they are carried away by the wind. After getting over their very hectic first day in a new home, Meg and Sarah sensibly decide to look for somewhere else to live.

## JONATHAN CREEK (2004)

Jonathan Creek is an English comedy drama series with the lead character being played by comedian, Alan Davies. Jonathan is a production assistant and deviser of intriguing illusions for magician, Adam Klaus's stage show. As such he finds that he is continually asked to solve impossible mysteries with his rapier-sharp mind that sees seemingly insignificant details which other people do not. In an episode set in the world of fashion design, *The Tailor's Dummy*, centres around the revelation that the elderly but highly acclaimed fashion designer, Marco Bergman, can no longer produce anything new. It is in fact his son, Claude and daughter, Louise (played by Maureen Lipman) who have been making all the decisions about what the latest trend or style would be.

A particularly acid-tongued reporter, Donna Henry, writes a bad review of Marco Bergman's latest designs, and Louise becomes obsessed with getting revenge. Much is made of how upset her father is by the vicious words Donna Henry has written. Louise devises a clever plan where she literally gets Donna Henry to eat her words when a gunman enters her hotel room and stands over her while she swallows her shredded magazine article. Unfortunately Marco Bergman later throws himself out of a third-floor bedroom window to his death, but not before he has also flung his parrot, Harvey, out too and made sure that his cage safely lands in the bushes below. It is assumed by everyone affected by the death that Bergman could not take the vicious criticism regarding his work any longer.

Claude's daughter, Carrie, comes to stay and Jonathan Creek receives a frantic phone call from her, urging him to come to the house immediately because she has been locked in her bedroom. Jonathan Creek, master of solving the sealed room mystery, arrives to find that Carrie has climbed out of a bedroom window in desperation and is standing on the ledge, three floors up, mimicking her grandfather's actions before his death. When Creek rushes inside the house, Louise is found shouting outside Carrie's locked bedroom door, trying to discern what is wrong with her niece. Finally, Louise locates the door key and Carrie is inside, pale and looking very anxious.

An earlier emphasis is made of the teenager rolling up her sleeve and selecting a syringe from her bag. Aunt Louise charges into the room and snatches the syringe away from the girl, intimating her disapproval at the Carrie's actions. When Creek and Louise enter the bedroom later, Carrie announces that her aunt is trying to kill her as she has taken away her insulin. When asked by Louise why she would deprive a diabetic of their medication, Carrie replies that it is because she (Carrie) knows. Presumably Carrie only brought one syringe with her on her visit, otherwise she could have drawn up a second dose and injected herself when her aunt had left the room.

As the storyline moves on it is revealed that Louise was tired of failing to get the recognition she felt she deserved for her work. In a very cruel way, Louise had decided to kill her father by staging a fire. Jonathan Creek works out that Marco Bergman was actually blind for the last couple of years of his life because there are scratches around the lock on his wardrobe door and because his socks are pinned together in pairs. Louise confirms this was the reason she and Claude took over the design aspect of her father's fashion empire. She emphasises that this was a secret that nobody could know because the famous Bergman designs would become worthless if they were not Marco Bergman originals.

Louise had recorded the sounds of an inferno on tape which would start to play when her father was sleeping. Marco Bergman was known to be terrified of fire after an experience of flying in a burning aircraft in the war. In the middle of the night (it is not explained where Claude was at this time), Louise shouts to her father that he must wake up as the whole floor is ablaze, and that his only chance of surviving the life-threatening flames is to jump from the third-floor window, where they had placed plenty of cushions for him to land on. The poor man had to go on trust that this information was true, and although there was no actual heat, his imagination filled in any gaps about the intensity of the fire that the tape could not conjure up.

Retrospectively the episode shows Carrie in the kitchen. She removes the rubbish bag and sees an audio tape lying in the bottom of the bin which she plays, finding on it the sounds of a crackling, raging fire. This is the reason her aunt had locked her in her room without insulin, because it would prevent Carrie from telling anyone what Louise had done. However, in reality it would take more than an hour without insulin to induce hyperglycaemia that led to a fatal coma. It is stated that if Louise's niece fell into a diabetic coma, no one would question this. This gives the impression that missing one insulin injection ultimately leads to death, and that no one would find that Carrie was locked in her bedroom (her father, for example, who also lived in the house). Carrie is not shown to be giving herself any insulin after she is released from the room.

Jonathan Creek sums up that Marco Bergman was trying to save his parrot by throwing his cage into the bushes, meaning that Bergman's death certainly was not due to suicide. As everyone present stares at Louise in horror and disbelief at what she has done, she is pleased with herself for her ingenuity, telling everyone how clever she has been. There is no sadness or guilt as she announces that she did it for Claude and herself as she was tired of her father's cold arrogance in not acknowledging her design genius. To Marco Bergman, Louise had only been "the perfect repository for his creations".

## Soap opera

A character with diabetes provides soap opera plot writers with the scope for all kinds of dramatic situations, but all too often reality is barely depicted. The following examples of portrayals of diabetes in a soap scenario are chosen because they are factually correct, although the situations surrounding them are sometimes rather far-fetched. The English soap, *Coronation Street*, is set in the cobbled backstreets of Weatherfield in Northern Manchester. Katy Harris, a girl in her mid-teens, began to feel thirsty and could not quench it, drinking full-sugar lemonade as she was unaware what was wrong with her. However, no other symptoms were depicted such as rapid weight loss, tiredness, or frequent urination due to hyperglycaemia.

Katy was helped to come to terms with the diagnosis of Type 1 diabetes and with injecting her insulin (although this would normally be the role of a diabetes nurse specialist) by general nurse and neighbour, Martin Platt, with whom she developed a close relationship although he was 20 years older than her. Katy later became pregnant, but her father, Tommy, persuaded her to get rid of the child, not because he was worried about his daughter's diabetes and how this would be affected by her pregnancy, but because he hated Martin Platt. Full of revenge, Katy went to the garage where her father worked and hit him over the head with a wrench, killing him instantly. This naturally caused family conflict and Katy's mother,

Angela, who had witnessed the murder, decided to take the blame on her daughter's behalf and was arrested for her husband's death.

After several months Katy could no longer stand the guilt of what she had done and began drinking sugar mixed with water, then eating sugar directly from the bag, eventually lapsing into a hyperglycaemic coma. She was found by Martin Platt and rushed to hospital, but she had suffered brain swelling (cerebral oedema), one of the major consequences of hyperglycaemic coma (British Society for Paediatric Endocrinology and Diabetes, 2009). This condition is associated with headache and a fluctuating level of consciousness in some patients and respiratory arrest in others. Cerebral oedema is the most common cause of mortality in children with diabetes and ketoacidosis, but less often in adolescents and young adults. Katy died shortly after her admission to hospital having never regained consciousness. This was her last appearance in April 2005.

The Australian soap, *Neighbours,* is set in the suburbs of Melbourne, with much of the action occurring on Ramsay Street. Danni (short for Danielle) Stark arrived in 1993 and was quickly labelled a trouble-maker when a resident of Ramsay Street saw Danni injecting herself with insulin and immediately assumed it was heroin, feeling the need to gossip about this. This assumption is often portrayed on screen when a syringe is taken out of a bag, and the accusation of being a drug addict has actually happened to the author when it was necessary to inject insulin (in a surreptitious way so as not to draw attention to the fact) in a public place with no bathroom facilities. This storyline also appears in the film, *Mad Money* (2009), where a man carrying insulin syringes in his bag is thought to be a heroin addict. Potential practical difficulties with having Type 1 diabetes were well-portrayed in one episode of *Neighbours* when Danni Stark and her boyfriend went away on holiday and found themselves caught up in a flood situation where they were stranded without food or water and she developed low blood glucose levels. This was depicted as anxiety, but other symptoms were not shown. Of course in reality, people who take insulin usually carry glucose or food in case of emergencies rather than walking around for hours, burning up even more glucose looking for food. This episode illustrates very well what can potentially happen when the individual is unprepared. Danni was portrayed as being angry at how life has treated her, and this rings true when a young person is having difficulty coming to terms with managing their chronic condition which marks them as different from their friends.

Although exceedingly headstrong, Danni was actually a talented young fashion designer, although she was also manipulative and enjoyed any attention. At a typically Australian pool party where all the young people in the neighbourhood had gathered, Danni decided, for dramatic effect, to have full-sugar soft drinks rather than her usual diet, sugar-free ones. Aided by hyperglycaemia making her thirsty due to the sugar in the drinks, Danni continued to gulp them down until her vision became blurry and she collapsed in a heap at the pool side. After hospitalisation, she recovered, but received several warnings about her stupidity. Danni's character was eventually written out of the series in November 1996.

*Emmerdale* is set in an English farming community. Character Kerry Wyatt is a person with Type 1 diabetes in her thirties, although she drinks heavily and does very little to look after her condition. As the peak incidence of Type 1 diabetes is in the teens, this assumes Kerry has had diabetes for at least ten years, although there is no portrayal of diabetic eye disease (retinopathy) or peripheral nerve damage in the feet which might be expected for someone with long-term erratic blood glucose management. Perhaps Kerry's haemoglobin A1c (the amount of glucose sticking to the red blood cells and triggering complications in excess) is kept low due to her alcoholism.

An episode portrayed Kerry getting very drunk and slipping into unconsciousness whilst she was meant to be childminding. The fact that she also smokes caused a fire as a lit cigarette was left to burn. Kerry was then admitted to hospital in a hypoglycaemic coma and the storyline attempted to highlight the seriousness of low blood glucose levels. Over forty years ago the International Broadcasting Authority stated that viewers absorbed medical information from soap opera scenarios more readily, especially if it is a character that they care about, than if facts were provided in a public information broadcast or health campaign. A further storyline focussed around Kerry's insulin pen being stolen by a child she was looking after, meaning Kerry did not take her insulin and went into a hyperglycaemic coma. When she was admitted to hospital, doctors decided Kerry was unconscious because she was drunk. This gave viewers conflicting information regarding hyperglycaemia and hypoglycaemia. The character of Kerry Wyatt was still current in 2014.

In Australian soap, *Home and Away,* the character of Ruby Buckton was portrayed for four years until 2012 as a promiscuous teenage schoolgirl who had Type 1 diabetes. Ruby was a binge-drinker with numerous emotional entanglements and problems that meant she did not look after her condition. Ruby's diabetes was only a minor storyline, and she went about her life with little attention to any diabetes self-management, being found unconscious, as is the usual soap depiction of a person with Type 1 diabetes, again due to the dangerous combination of alcohol-induced hypoglycaemia and insulin. This attitude did demonstrate to viewers the dangers faced by adolescents who chose to ignore their diabetes, which sadly does happen as seen in the denial of the seriousness of managing blood glucose levels in diabulimia. As with all depictions of diabetes in soap opera, the emphasis is on the drama of the situation rather than any educational opportunity, but it is hoped that viewers remember the fictitious situations they have seen and take from this something positive about the condition and its management.

## BOOKS

Two television adaptations based on stories by Agatha Christie have already been discussed concerning one death assisted by insulin and one person with diabetes who was killed with insulin after consuming alcohol. These depictions were included because Christie had background knowledge of how insulin can kill. The drama of hyperglycaemic coma, often portrayed in soap opera, is also depicted in fiction books in the same way, only there is more scope for detail: the youngster with diabetes who has difficulty coming to terms with their condition, not seeing the danger in combining insulin and large quantities of alcohol, or that by ignoring Type 1 diabetes, it tends to come back and hit hard in a medical emergency. Such a depiction in book format is that of 16-year old Lucy Szabo in *Sweetblood* by Pete Hautman (2010), where her condition leads to frequent hyperglycaemia, and a very true-to-life description of ketoacidosis.

*Sweetblood* is aimed at the teenage reader, with a clever storyline where Lucy has researched the subject of vampirism in legend and concludes that the reason for their reported uncontrollable thirst and deathly pallor was due to Type 1 diabetes. This is also alluded to in the film *Blade* (1998) where a charred body is brought to a hospital morgue and the autopsy reveals that the corpse's blood glucose level is three times the normal amount shortly before the body, an undead vampire, attacks the two people dissecting him. Whilst this idea might be somewhat far-fetched, *Sweetblood* is particularly good in bringing the reality of managing adolescent diabetes, with its hormonal variations and blood glucose management difficulties, to the page in a way that television does not have time to accommodate.

There are a number of books which briefly mention a character with diabetes, or a hypoglycaemic episode, but not in any great detail because they are not books about diabetes, meaning few actually base the whole story around a character with the condition, depicting their struggles and victories. In *True Believers* (2013) by Kurt Anderson, the eminent attorney, Karen Hollander, now in her mid-60s is depicted as having Type 1 diabetes from childhood. The storyline concerns the fact that Karen is writing her memoirs, revealing her revolutionary acts and secrets during the 1960s. Karen keeps herself fit and is a very slim American size 6, although she does mention taking hallucinogenic drugs as she looks back on her past, but does not describe whether this affected her blood glucose levels. This story shows that Type 1 diabetes need not be restrictive in terms of having an extremely successful career.

In the Kurt Wallander series of books by Henning Mankell, the seventh book describes Wallader developing Type 2 diabetes, a rare change from the usually-depicted Type 1 which gives more scope for hypoglycaemia and ketoacidosis storylines. In *One Step Behind* (2012), the symptoms of Type 2 diabetes, which is of much slower onset than Type 1, are depicted as Wallander becomes increasingly thirsty and then needs to urinate more often: typical symptoms of the condition which hopefully serve to be educational to the reader. The book also shows that Wallander is able to control his condition reasonably well by paying attention to his diet and taking regular exercise, meaning he is able to handle his career as a detective. This demonstrates that diabetes does not have to define the individual, but that a balance must be struck so that the condition is recognised and managed.

# Glossary of Terms

Absolute insulin deficiency: the result of the development of Type 1 diabetes or due to lack of administration of insulin.

Acini: masses of cells surrounding the Islets of Langerhans in the pancreas which secrete digestive enzymes.

Acromegaly: a condition typified by over-production of growth hormone by the pituitary gland, leading to excessive height and associated heath problems.

A.D.A.: American Diabetes Association.

Adipocytes: fat cells where glucose is stored as triglycerides.

Adrenaline (epinephrine): released by the adrenal glands in response to stress, increasing the rate of respiration, heart rate, and improving muscle performance in the fight or flight response.

Alanine: a non-carbon substrate generated by the liver to produce glucose.

Alpha blockers: drugs used to treat high blood pressure.

Alpha cells: found in the Islets of Langerhans and producing the hormone glucagon which raises blood glucose levels.

Amlodipine: a medication used to block calcium uptake which can increase blood glucose levels.

Amphetamines: drugs similar to adrenaline which stimulate the central nervous system and induce a feeling of well-being and alertness; they also cause an increased heart rate and are highly addictive.

Anabolic androgenic steroids: are produced from derivatives of testosterone, the male hormone produced in the testes from puberty in both females and males, although females also produce around 10 percent of the level seen in males.

Anabolic metabolism (anabolism): the production of larger molecules from smaller ones.

Angiography: a method of scanning the heart and arteries and treating blockages in these vessels.

Anorexia: a disorder where there is an obsessive fear of gaining weight resulting in severe dietary restriction.

Anti-diuretic hormone (ADH): a hormone which inhibits the production of urine and helps adrenaline (also known as epinephrine) and glucose increase blood glucose levels.

A.P.A.: American Psychiatric Association.

Aphasia: errors when speaking.

Atenolol: a beta blocker medication for high blood pressure which can raise blood glucose levels.

Atrophy: wasting of a body part, usually due to lack of use, malnutrition or ageing, but also associated with taking anabolic androgenic steroids, associated with atrophy of the testes.

Atracurium besylate: a skeletal muscle relaxant used during surgical procedures and mechanical ventilation.

Autoacids: the term used by Sir Edward Schafer in 1916 in reference to the stimulating actions of insulin on other processes in the body.

Autoimmune attack: the body's defence mechanism. Type 1 diabetes is an autoimmune disease where the body attacks its own insulin-producing beta cells in the pancreas.

Autoimmune syndrome: a condition resulting in a high concentration of insulin in the blood despite low blood glucose levels.

Autonomic nervous system: the nervous system controlling automatic bodily functions which are not conscious actions such as cardiovascular, gastrointestinal, genitourinary, metabolic and sub-motor function.

Autonomic neuropathy: damage to the autonomic nerves controlling involuntary functions such as digestion and cardiac functions.

Babinski reflex test: to test for the level and stage of brain function in comatose patients, this reflex usually occurs in response to stroking the outer margin of the sole of the foot, where the big toe will move downwards if there is no neurological impairment and upwards if there is impairment present.

Barbiturates: sedatives which lower blood pressure, body temperature, and depress the central nervous system and respiration.

Basal ganglia: the area of the brain responsible for translating our memories into motivation, motor selection and action, controlling large and small muscle movement.

Bezafibrate: a fibric acid derivative drug used to treat disorders of fat.

Beta blockers: drugs used to treat high blood pressure.

Beta cells: found in the Islets of Langerhans and producing the hormone insulin which lowers blood glucose levels.

Biological antagonism: a term coined by the Hungarian physician, Meduna in 1933 meaning that one medical condition (schizophrenia) could not fully manifest its symptoms in the presence of another (epilepsy).

Bisopropol: a beta blocker medication for high blood pressure which can raise blood glucose levels.

Body dysmorphia: a condition where the individual has an unrealistic, negative view of their body and how they appear to others.

Brain cortex: responsible for our choice of correct social behaviour, higher thinking, planning, reasoning, judgement, self-regulation, and impulse control.

Bronchodilators: inhaled drugs taken by people with asthma to increase the size of their airway, but also abused by body builders in order to exploit their effect of reducing the amount of fat and fluid in the muscle tissue.

Bulimia: a disorder characterised by binge eating, then vomiting or laxative abuse.

Cannula: a small tube used for medical purposes.

Catecholamine: are substances produced by the adrenal glands in response to stress, triggering the release of glucagon by the liver.

Catabolism: chemical reactions that break down complex organic compounds into simple ones with the release of energy.

Cataract: cloudiness of the lens of the eye.

Cardiac arrhythmia: an alteration in the normal heart rhythm.

Cardiomyopathy: a serious condition of the heart and circulatory system thought to stem from damage to the autonomic nerves controlling parts of the body not under conscious control, for example, the heartbeat.

C.B.T. (Cognitive Behavioural Therapy): is a psychotherapeutic therapy addressing dysfunctional emotional patterns, maladaptive behaviours, and cognitive processes using goal-driven systematic methods.

Cerebral oedema: swelling of the brain.

Cerebrovascular accident: stroke.

Chalones: a term used by Sir Edward Schafer in 1916 in reference to the inhibitory actions of insulin on certain body processes.

Charcot foot: a chronic complication of diabetes which refers to the degeneration of the joints of the foot due to nerve damage, loss of sensation, and excess areas of pressure.

Chlorpromazine: an anti-psychotic medication which can increase blood glucose levels.

Clofibrate: a fibric acid derivative drug used to treat disorders of fat.

Cognitive impairment: the alteration of normal thought processes and patterns.

Compliance: concerns the idea that the individual should do what they are told by health professionals.

Complications (chronic) of diabetes: hyperglycaemia leads to eye disease (retinopathy); kidney disease (nephropathy); nerve damage (neuropathy); microvascular disease (affecting small blood vessels); macrovascular disease (affecting the heart and arteries); and stroke.

Cortisol: a hormone released by the adrenal glands when we are stressed which raises blood glucose levels and suppresses the immune system and slows digestion.

C-peptide: is an essential but biologically inactive building block of insulin formed during the manufacture of insulin by the beta cells of the pancreas.

C.T. scan: Computed Tomography scan using x-rays.

Creatine (phosphate): a high-energy molecule in the cells of skeletal muscle fibre that quickly generate adenosine triphosphate (ATP), breaking down into creatine, phosphate, and energy.

Creutzfeldt-Jakob disease: a condition also known as spongiform encephalopathy, causing rapid deterioration of the brain and progressive dementia.

Cyclosporine: a drug used to prevent rejection after organ transplant surgery which can also increase blood glucose levels.

Cytoplasm: the jelly-like substance surrounding the nucleus of a cell.

Delta cells: found in the Islets of Langerhans and producing growth hormone-inhibiting hormone, also known as somastostatin.

Diabulimia: the practice by some people (particularly adolescent females) with Type 1 diabetes of deliberately omitting or giving a low dose of insulin to induce ketoacidosis in order to achieve rapid weight loss.

Diaphoresis: profuse sweating.

Degradation: a term relating to the breakdown of a used insulin molecule by the cells which has used the insulin.

Dextrose: another name for glucose, known as D-glucose.

Doxazosin: a drug known as an alpha-blocker, used to treat high blood pressure.

E.E.G.: electroencephalograph, a measure of brain activity.

E.S.R.D. (End-Stage Renal Disease): kidney failure.

Endocrine gland: a ductless gland that secretes hormones into the bloodstream.

Epiphyses: growth plates in the long bones of the arms and legs which disappear when the bones stop growing and the head and shaft of the bones fuse.

Ergometrine: an abortion-inducing drug.

Etomidate: a short-acting intravenous anaesthetic used to render a patient anaesthetised or sedated for procedures such as relocating dislocated joints.

Exocrine gland: a gland that secretes hormones into ducts that empty into epithelial tissue or directly into a body cavity.

Exogenous: injected insulin rather than insulin produced by the pancreas.

F-cells: found in the Islets of Langerhans and producing a polypeptide to regulate the release of the pancreatic digestive enzymes amylase, trypsin and lipase.

Factitious insulin-induced hypoglycaemia: insulin that is injected by either the individual or someone else for the purposes of gaining attention or sympathy.

Fasting hypoglycaemia: a condition where blood glucose levels are low due to inadequate stores of glycogen (such as when dieting) or due to slow conversion of glycogen into glucose when needed. The condition may also be brought about by the consumption of alcohol, and by breast or adrenal cancer.

Fibric acid derivatives: drugs used to treat disorders of fat.

Fibroblasts: large, flat cells forming collagen and elastic fibres and intercellular substances in connective tissue.

Fluphenazine: an anti-psychotic medication which can increase blood glucose levels.

Frontal lobe (also see brain cortex): the anterior part of the cerebral hemisphere of the cerebrum of the brain. It creates our personality and is the emotional centre of the brain responsible for empathy, decision making, problem solving, judgement, impulses, and self-regulation.

Frontal lobotomy (also see psychosurgery): surgically severing the connections between the prefrontal cortex and the underlying structures of the brain, or completely destroying the frontal cortex tissue.

Fructose: fruit sugars.

Galactosaemia: a rare condition seen in children where the ability to process galactose (natural sugars found in milk) is impaired.

Galactose: milk sugars.

Game theory: how chance governs the systems used in daily life.

Gastroparesis: damage to the nerves controlling the rate of digestion, resulting in delayed stomach emptying and slow digestive transit. This condition results in difficulty matching insulin dosages to rates of digestion, leading to hypo- and hyperglycaemia.

Gestational diabetes: a condition similar to Type 2 diabetes which develops from the $20^{th}$ week of pregnancy.

Ghrelin: a substance produced by the parietal cells of the stomach in response to fasting to promote a sensation of hunger.

Glucagon: a substance which attaches to the liver cells to make them release stored glucose quickly.

Glycogenesis: the conversion of excess glucose into glycogen for storage in the liver.

Gluconeogenesis: the metabolic pathway resulting in the generation of glucose from non-carbohydrate sources such as amino acids, glycerol or lactic acid, enabling the release of glucose into the body.

Glycaemic control: maintaining blood glucose levels between 4.0–7.0mmol/L (72–126mg/dl).

Glycogen: a form of glucose stored in the liver cells.

Glycogenolysis: a process accelerated by glycogen whereby stored glucose in the liver is converted into usable glucose to raise blood glucose levels.

Glycogen storage disease: a condition where the enzyme which breaks down stored glycogen into glucose sub-units is faulty causing slow release of glucose by the liver and resulting hypoglycaemia.

Glycolysis: the process by which glucose is converted into pyruvic acid, a ketone acid.

Glucoregulation: how the body responds to glucose.

Glycerol: a simple sugar and alcohol compound.

Goitre: a swelling in the neck due to enlargement of the thyroid gland when production of thyroid hormones is increased. This may occur due to a lack of dietary iodine (endemic or simple goitre), or due to auto-immune disease (hyperplasia).

Gonadotrophin: hormones produced by the pituitary gland. Follicle-stimulating hormone is produced in both males and females to control directly or indirectly the growth of the ova and sperm; as is luteinising hormone which stimulates reproductive activity in the gonads.

Graves disease: a condition whereby the thyroid gland is over-active.

Grey matter: part of the central nervous system comprising the central part of the spinal cord, the cerebral cortex, and the outer layer of the cerebellum in the brain. It is the co-ordination point between the nerves of the central nervous system.

Growth hormone: a substance produced by the anterior pituitary gland, the amount of which is controlled by growth hormone releasing hormone and growth hormone inhibiting hormone.

Growth hormone deficiency disease: a condition causing hypoglycaemia because growth hormone restricts the action of insulin on muscle and fat cells leading to increased sensitivity to insulin, forcing the pancreas to produce more insulin.

Gynecomastia: the development of breast tissue in males, a common side effect of taking anabolic androgenic steroids.

Haemofiltration: dialysis.

Haemolysis: a state where the red blood cells burst in a blood sample, making it useless for insulin for C-peptide analysis.

Hallux rigidus: dislocation of the big toe joint.

Hashish: dried hemp used for smoking or chewing.

HbA1c: the amount of glucose sticking to the red blood cells over a three-month period measured to determine control of blood glucose levels.

Hepatic: liver.

Hereditary fructose disorder: a condition causing hypoglycaemia in children because the body cannot metabolise natural fruit sugar.

Hippocampus: a region of the brain which works quickly to locate and retrieve memories.

Homeostasis: the control and balance of body energy in humans.

Hyperglycaemia: high blood glucose levels of >13mmol/L (234 mg/dl).

Hyperinsulinaemic clamp: a process used by athletes to boost muscle building by exploiting the action of injected insulin, offsetting its blood glucose-lowering effects by eating high-carbohydrate foods to avoid hypoglycaemia.

Hyperinsulinism: the over-production of insulin.

Hypertension: high blood pressure in the arteries. Essential hypertension may be due to an unknown cause such as kidney failure or endocrine disease.

Hyperthyroidism: an over-active thyroid gland producing too much thyroxin.

Hypoglycaemia: low blood glucose levels of <4.0mmol/L (<72mg/dl).

Hypoglycaemic encephalopathy: disease (death of areas of cells) of the brain brought about by very low blood glucose levels.

Hypothalamic: pertaining to the hypothalamus region of the brain, controlling fat and carbohydrate metabolism, thirst and fluid regulation, appetite, temperature regulation, and sexual function. The hypothalamus is also involved with our emotions and the regulation of sleep, controls the sympathetic and parasympathetic nervous systems, and secretions from the pituitary gland.

Hypothermia: a reduction of the core body temperature to below 35 degrees centigrade.

Hypothyroidism: an underactive thyroid gland which produces too little thyroxin.

Hypoxia: a prolonged reduction in oxygen.

Immuran: a drug used to prevent rejection after organ transplant surgery which can also increase blood glucose levels.

Insulin: a polypeptide hormone (a chemical messenger) and a protein produced by the beta cells of the pancreas.

Insulin coma treatment (also known as insulin shock treatment): a treatment developed in the 1930s for schizophrenia, psychosis and addiction involving injecting large doses of insulin into patients to achieve a comatose state with severe hypoglycaemia.

Insulin Detemir: a brand of long-acting insulin.

Insulin Glargine: a brand of long-acting insulin.

Insulin-like growth factor: a small protein produced in response to human growth hormone by the liver, chondrocytes (cells of mature cartilage), and skeletal muscle fibres which stimulate growth. It also acts as an indicator for the action of growth hormone on the liver.

Insulinoma: an insulin-secreting tumour, usually benign.

Insulin hyperplasia: a rare condition where there is enlargement of the insulin-producing beta cells of the pancreases causing frequent hypoglycaemia due to excess insulin.

Insulin pump (also known as Continuous Subcutaneous Insulin Infusion): a method of delivering a continual basal rate of insulin under the skin with measured dosages for meals and at times when additional insulin is required.

Insulin resistance: inability of body cells to use insulin correctly to reduce blood glucose levels, causing the pancreas to produce even more insulin.

Insulin sensitivity: the ability of body cells to use insulin correctly to reduce blood glucose levels.

Islet hyperplasia: a condition where the alpha islet cells producing glucagon and the beta islet cells producing insulin are uniformly enlarged because of an increase in the number of alpha cells.

Islets of Langerhans: two to three million tiny clusters of hormone-producing cells found in the exocrine tissue of the pancreas.

J.D.R.F.: Juvenile Diabetes Research Foundation.

Ketoacidosis: a severe metabolic imbalance where there is a breakdown of fats as an alternative source of energy to glucose that cannot be used when there is a lack of insulin. This results in the production of acid by-products which, in large quantities, create a medical emergency.

Ketogenesis: the process where ketone bodies are formed due to fatty acid breakdown.

Ketones: the waste products of protein metabolism.

Lantus: a brand of long-acting insulin.

Leptin: is an appetite suppressant produced by the adipose (fatty) tissue during sleep.

Levemir: a brand of long-acting insulin.

Lipogenesis: the conversion of glucose and other nutrients into fatty acids.

Lipolysis: the regulation of protein synthesis and the mobilisation of fat controlled by growth hormone.

Macrovascular disease: refers to heart and artery disease.

Melatonin: a hormone produced by the pineal gland, the action of which suppresses libido in accordance with the fight or flight response by reducing luteinizing hormone and follicle stimulating hormone secretion by the anterior pituitary gland.

Metabolism: the way the body uses energy to maintain its functions.

Methamphetamine: a powerful stimulant.

Metrazol: a drug which, when injected, rapidly causes seizures similar to epileptic fits. Used by Hungarian physician, Meduna in the 1930s to induce fits in patients as a treatment for schizophrenia.

Modafinil: prescribed as a mild stimulant for the condition of narcolepsy, where individuals continually and spontaneously fall asleep for very short periods throughout the day.

Microalbuminuria: minute amounts of albumin in the urine, albumin being the smallest and most abundant plasma protein, which maintains osmotic pressure. This is the first sign that diabetic kidney disease (nephropathy) is developing due to persistent hyperglycaemia.

Microvascular disease: damage to the small blood vessels.

Minoxidil: a powerful medication used to treat high blood pressure which can raise blood glucose levels.

Myocardial infarction: heart attack.

M.R.I.: Magnetic Resonance Imaging scan which does not use x-rays.

N.E.D.A.: National Eating Disorders Association.

N.R.E.M.: non-rapid eye movement sleep.

Nephropathy: a condition caused by hyperglycaemia where the nephrons of the kidney are damaged, impairing function. It is defined as a persistent and clinically detectable level of protein in the urine in association with an elevated blood pressure and reduced kidney function.

Nesidioblastosis: a rare disorder characterised by the secretion of large amounts of insulin and C-peptide in children, but also high blood glucose levels.

Neuropathy: damage to the central or peripheral nerves, or both. Peripheral neuropathy is a chronic complication of diabetes which occurs in two types: diffuse neuropathy, commonly appearing as disorders of sensation in the extremities of the body, and distal polyneuropathy, affecting many nerves of the hands and feet.

Neuropsychiatric: pertaining to the nervous system and brain.

Nicotinic acid (niacin): vitamin B3 prescribed in a high dosage to lower cholesterol levels which can increase blood glucose levels.

Nifedipine: a medication used to block calcium uptake which can raise blood glucose levels.

Nephropathy: is a chronic complication of diabetes caused by persistently high blood glucose levels leading to hardening of the kidney tissue and changes in the structure of the tubular epithelial cells of the kidneys.

Non-concordance: the action of an individual in choosing not to stick to a health care plan agreed between the individual and their health care professional. This term superseded the term "non-compliance".

Normoglycaemia: maintaining blood glucose levels within the normal range of 4.0–7.0mmol/L (72–126mg/dl).

O.S.A.: Obstructive Sleep Apnea is a condition causing intermittent and continual cessation of breathing leading to reduced levels of oxygen in the blood.

Octreotide: a drug which blocks the secretion of insulin by the pancreas, used to determine an insulin-producing tumour.

Osmotic diuresis: the production of urine.

Osmotic pressure: fluid balance inside and outside body cells.

Pancreatic amylase: an enzyme produced by the pancreas to break downs starchy foods.

Pancreatic lipase: an enzyme produced by the pancreas to break down triglycerides into fatty acids.

Parietal cells: cells in the stomach which produce hydrochloric acid to aid digestion.

Phosphorylase: the enzyme which breaks down glucose into sub-units.

Pilocarpine: a constituent of eye drops which causes the ciliary muscles in the eyes to contract. Pilocarpine is also an antidote to atropine poisoning.

Prednisone: a drug used to prevent rejection after organ transplant surgery which can also increase blood glucose levels.

Prevalence: refers to the pattern of occurrence of a disease.

Pro-insulin: the molecule from which insulin is made by the beta cells of the pancreas.

Promazine: an anti-psychotic medication which can increase blood glucose levels.

Proteases: substances that break down proteins.

Proteolysis: a process where protein is synthesised and broken down to be used as fuel when glucose cannot be metabolised.

Psychosurgery (also see frontal lobotomy): the selective surgical removal of destructive nerve pathways or normal brain tissue with a view to influencing behaviour.

Pulmonary oedema: congestion of the lungs.

R.E.M.: rapid eye movement sleep.

Radioimmunoassay: a technique using radioactive insulin and antibody studies able to measure tiny amounts of insulin, reacting only with the antibody, in blood and tissues. This has now been superseded by mass spectrometry techniques.

Reactive hypoglycaemia: a reduction in blood glucose level due to the body producing too much insulin.

Recombinant: substances artificially manufactured in the laboratory, such as insulin or growth hormone.

Renal: kidney.

Relative insulin deficiency: a consequence of under-dosing on insulin or a failure to meet metabolic need.

Respiratory acidosis: a condition whereby decreased oxygen intake leads to a build up of carbon dioxide in the blood, reducing cell and tissue acidity to below 7.35 pH.

Retinopathy: a chronic complication of diabetes which describes a number of symptoms including abnormal dilation of the blood vessels of the eyes and haemorrhages of the retina. In advanced cases the retina becomes heavily scarred and may lead to blindness.

Sakel Technique: insulin coma treatment for mental illness invented by Dr Manfred Sakel.

Salicylates: aspirin and drugs derived from aspirin.

Schizophrenia: a severe personality disorder with symptoms including hallucinations, delusions, blunted emotions, disordered thinking, and a withdrawal from reality.

Scoliosis: un-natural curvature of the spine.

Septicaemia: blood poisoning.

Serotonin: a hormone which gives us a sense of wellbeing.

Shift work disorder: hormonal imbalance seen in people who work at night and sleep during the day.

Slow-wave sleep: the third and fourth part of a 90-minute cycle of non-rapid eye movement sleep.

Somastostatin: also known as growth hormone-inhibiting hormone.

Subcutaneous: under the skin.

Tacrolimus: a drug used to prevent rejection after organ transplant surgery which can also increase blood glucose levels.

Testosterone: the male sex hormone which stimulates the production of sperm and the development and maintenance of the appearance of male characteristics.

Tetrahydrogestrinone: a designer anabolic steroid substance.

Thebain: an opiate and class A drug similar to morphine and codeine.

Theobromine: an alkaloid found in tea, chocolate and cocoa beverages which is poisonous to humans at a level of 300mg per kilogram of body-weight.

Thermoregulation: control of body temperature.

Thiazide: diuretics which can raise blood glucose levels by increasing the amount of potassium lost in the urine.

Thioridazine: an anti-psychotic medication (not now used in the UK) which can increase blood glucose levels.

Thyroxin: a hormone produced by the thyroid gland which is essential for the regulation of metabolism and growth.

Thyrotoxicosis: an over-active thyroid gland.

Tolbutamide: a drug used to stimulate the pancreas to produce insulin during a glucose tolerance test.

Triiodothyronine: a hormone produced by the thyroid gland which is essential for the regulation of metabolism and growth.

Triglycerides: blood fats.

Tripfluoperzaine: an anti-psychotic medication which can increase blood glucose levels.

Trypsin: an enzyme produced by the pancreas to break down protein.

Type 1 diabetes: a condition where the pancreatic beta cells do not produce insulin, or only a very small amount, due to auto-immune attack on the insulin-producing cells triggered by a virus.

Type 2 diabetes: a condition where there is an over-production of insulin produced because it cannot be used effectively if there is excess body fat impeding its function on cells.

Vasopressin: a hormone released by the liver with adrenaline and glucagon to help raise blood glucose levels when they are low. It also encourages human pair bonding, attachment and monogamy, and reduces aggression in males.

Vitreous humour: a jelly-like substance found between lens and the retina of the eye.

# References

Abrams R (1988) *Electroconvulsive Therapy.* Oxford: Oxford University Press.

Ackard DM, Neumark-Sztainer VN, Schmitz KH, et al (2008) Disordered eating and body dissatisfaction in adolescents with Type 1 diabetes and a population-based comparison sample: comparative prevalence and clinical implications. *Pediatric Diabetes* 9: 312–319.

Aimaretti G, Cornell G, Razzore C, et al (1998) Comparison between insulin-induced hypoglycaemia and growth hormone (GH)-releasing hormone + argentine as provocative tests for the diagnosis of GH deficiency in adults. *Journal of Clinical Endocrinology and Metabolism* 83(5): 1615–1618.

Alexander FG & Selesnick ST (1966). *The History of Psychiatry: An Evaluation of Psychiatric Thought and Practice from Prehistoric Times to the Present.* New York: Harper & Row.

Alonso-Vale MIC, Andreotti S, Peres SB, et al (2005) Melatonin enhances leptin expression by rat adipocytes in the presence of insulin. *American Journal of Physiology* 288(4): E805–E812.

American Diabetes Association www.diabetes.org

Amiel SA, Sherwin DC, Simonson AA, et al (1986) Impaired insulin action in puberty: a contributing factor to poor glycaemic control in adolescents with diabetes. *New England Journal of Medicine* 315(4): 215–219.

Anderson K (2013) *True Believers.* New York: Random House Trade.

Anderson RJ, Freeland KE, Clouse RE, et al (2001) The prevalence of comorbid depression in adults with diabetes: a meta-analysis. *Diabetes Care* 24: 1069–1078.

Anderson RM, Donnelly MB, Gressard CP (1989) Development of a diabetes attitude scale for health professionals. *Diabetes Care* 12: 120–127.

Anderson RM & Gressard CP (1987) Developing a measure of attitudes of healthcare providers towards diabetes and its treatment. *Diabetes Care* 36: 120A.

Arvanitakis C, Chen GH, Folscroft J, et al (1977) Effect of aspirin on intestinal absorption of glucose, sodium, and water in man. *Gut* 18, 187–190.

Askill J & Sharpe M (1993) *The Angel of Death.* London: Michael O'Mara Books.

Asvoid BO, Sandt T, Hestad K, et al (2010) Cognitive function in Type 1 diabetes with early exposure to severe hypoglycaemia. *Diabetes Care* 33: 1945–1947.

Auer RN (2004a) Hypoglycaemic brain damage. *Metabolic Brain Disease* 19: 169–175.

Auer RN (2004b) Hypoglycaemic brain damage. *Forensic Science International* 146: 105–110.

Austin EJ & Deary IJ (1999) Effects of repeated hypoglycaemia on cognitive function. *Diabetes Care* 22: 1273–1277.

Ayas NT, White DP, Al-Delaimy WK, et al (2003) A prospective study of self-reported sleep duration and incident diabetes in women. *Diabetes Care* 26(2): 280–284.

Bamberger M & Yaeger D (1997) Over the edge. *Sports Illustrated* 14: 62–70.

Banadonna RC, Saccomani MP, Cobelli C, et al (1993) Effect of insulin on system A amino acid transport on human skeletal muscle. *Journal of Clinical Investigation* 91: 514–521.

Bandura A (1977) Self-efficacy: towards a unifying theory of behaviour change. *Psychological Review* 84: 191–215.

Banting FG & Best CH (1922) The internal secretion of the pancreas. *Journal of Laboratory and Clinical Medicine* 7, 251–266.

Banting FG (1929) The history of insulin. *Edinburgh Medical Journal* 36, 1–18.

Barnett AH & Grice J (2011) *New Mechanisms in Glucose Control.* Chichester, West Sussex: John Wiley and Co. Limited.

Barraclough BM & Mitchell-Heggs NA (1974) Use of neurosurgery for psychological disorder in the British Isles during 1974–1976. *British Medical Journal* 2(6152): 1591–1593.

Basaria S, Wahlstrom JT, Dobs AS (2001) Anabolic androgenic steroid therapy in the treatment of chronic diseases. *Journal of Clinical Endocrinology and Metabolism* 86: 5108–5117.

Bauman WA & Yalow RS (1981) Insulin as a lethal weapon. *Journal of Forensic Science* 26: 594–598.

Bayliss WM & Starling EH (1902) The mechanism of pancreatic secretion. *Journal of Physiology* 28, 325–353.

Beckenstein N (1939) Results of Metrazol therapy in schizophrenia. *Psychiatric Quarterly* 13(1): 106–113.

Becker MH (1974) *The Health Belief Model and Personal Health Behaviour.* London: Charles B. Slack, Thorofare.

Bell GI, Pictet RL, Rutter WJ, et al (1980) Sequence of the human insulin gene. *Nature* 284(5751): 26–32.

Benedict C, Brede S, Schiöth HB, et al (2010) Intranasal insulin enhances postprandial thermogenesis and lowers postprandal serum insulin levels in healthy men. *Diabetes* 60(1): 114–118.

Benedict C, Hallscmid M, Hatke A, et al (2004) Intranasal insulin improves memory in humans. *Psychneuroendocrinology* 29(10): 1326–1334.

Berson SA & Yalow RS (1966) Insulin in blood and insulin antibodies. *The American Journal of Medicine* 40(5): 676–690.

Birkinshaw VJ, Gurr MR, Randall SS, et al (1958) Investigations in a case of murder by insulin poisoning. *British Medical Journal* ii: 463–468.

Brebbia DR & Altzhuler KZ (1965) Oxygen consumption rate and electroencephalographs stage of sleep *Science* 150(3703): 1621–1623.

Bree AJ, Puente EC, Dorit D-I, et al (2009) Diabetes increases brain damage caused by severe hypoglycaemia. *American Journal of Physiology, Endocrinology and Metabolism* 297: E194–E201.

Bridges PK & Bartlett JR (1977) Psychosurgery: Yesterday and today. *British Journal of Psychiatry* 131: 249–260.

British Broadcasting Corporation News (2013) Rebecca Leighton: Nurse suspended for stealing drugs. England: BBC, February 27, 2013.

British Society for Paediatric Endocrinology and Diabetes (2009) *Guidelines for the Management of DKA*. BSPED, Bristol.

Brooks B, Cistulli PA, Borkman M, et al (1994) Obstructive sleep apnea in obese noninsulin-dependent diabetic patients: effect of continuous positive airway pressure treatment on insulin responsiveness. *Journal of Endocrinology and Clinical Metabolism* 79(6): 1681–1685.

Brown P, Tompkins C, Juul S, et al (1978) Mechanisms of action of insulin in diabetic patients: a dose-related effect on glucose production and utilisation. *British Medical Journal* 1: 1239–1242.

Burns RB (1991) *Essential Psychology*. Massachusetts, USA: Kluwer Academic Publishers.

Butterfield GE, Thompson J, Rennie MJ, et al (1997) Effect of rhGH and rhIGF-1 treatment on protein utilization in elderly women. *American Journal of Physiology* 272: E94–E99.

Butch B, Keyes R, Clark S (2004) Pumps used to deliver lethal doses of etomidate and atracurium. *American Journal of Forensic Medicine and Pathology* 25(2): 159–160.

Carter H (2012) Steeping Hill hospital nurse bailed. London: The Guardian newspaper, January 12, 2012.

Cavaco B, Uchigata Y, Porto T, et al (2001) Hypoglycaemia due to insulin autoimmune syndrome: report of two cases with characterisation of HLA alleles and insulin antibodies. *European Journal of Endocrinology* 145(3): 311–316.

Chow J & Chow C (2007) *Hypoglycaemia for Dummies*. Second edition, London: John Wiley and Sons.

Christie A (1939) *Murder is Easy.*Collins Crime Club.

Christie A (1925) The case of the missing will. *Blue Book Magazine* 40(3).

Clark M (2003) Identification and treatment of depression in people with diabetes. *Diabetes and Primary Care* 5(3): 124–127.

Cleveland Clinic (2011) *DSM IV-TR Criteria for Eating Disorders* http://www.clevelandclinicmeded.com/medicalpubs/diseasemanagement/psychiatry-psychology/eating-disorders

Coghlan A (2001) Athletes may be increasingly using insulin. http://www.newscientist.com/news/news.jsp?id=ns99991129

Cohen LH, Novick RG, Ettleson A (1942) Frontal lobotomy in the treatment of chronic psychotic overactivity: report of six cases. *Psychosomatic Medicine* 4(1): 94–104.

Colago A, Cuocolo A, Marzullo P, et al (2001) Is the acromegalic cardiomyopathy reversible? Effect of 5-year normalization of growth hormone and insulin-like growth factor-1 levels on cardiac performance. *Journal of Clinical Endocrinology and Metabolism* 86: 1551–1557.

Colas C, Mathieu P, Tchbroutsky G (1991) Eating disorders and retinal lesions in type 1 (insulin-dependent) women (Letter). *Diabetologia* 34: 288.

Cole-Lewis H & Kershaw T (2010) Text messaging as a tool for behavioural change in disease prevention and management. *Epidemiology Review* 32(1): 56–69.

Colton PA, Olmstead M, Daneman D, et al (2007) Five-year prevalence and persistence of disturbed eating behaviour and eating disorders in girls with type 1 diabetes. *Diabetes Care* 30(11): 2861–2862.

Colton PA, Olmstead M, Daneman D, et al (2004) Disturbed eating behaviour and eating disorders in preteen and early teenage girls with type 1 diabetes: a case-controlled study. *Diabetes Care* 27(7): 1654–1659.

Comi G (1997) Evoked potentials in diabetes mellitus. *Clinical Neuroscience* 4: 374–379.

Copeland J, Peters R, Dillon P (2000) Anabolic androgenic steroid use disorders among a sample of Australian competitive and recreational users. *Drug and Alcohol Dependence* 60: 91–96.

Coughlin SR, Mawdsley L, Murgaza JA, et al (2007) Cardiovascular and metabolic effects of CPAP in obese males with OSA. *European Respiratory Journal* 29(4): 720–727.

Cournot M, Ruidavets J-B, Marquié J-C, et al (2004) Environmental factors associated with body mass index in a population of Southern France. *European Journal of Cardiovascular Prevention and Rehabilitation* 11(4): 291–297.

Crampin AC, Lamagni TL, Hope VD (1998) The risk of infection with HIV and hepatitis B in individuals who inject steroids in England and Wales. *Epidemiology Infection* 2: 381–386.

Cranston I (2005) Diabetes and the Brain. In: Shaw KM and Cummings MH (eds) *Diabetes Chronic Complications*. Second edition. Chichester, West Sussex: John Wiley & Sons Limited.

Criego A & Jahraus J (2009) Eating disorders and diabetes. *Diabetes Spectrum* 22(3): 135–136.

Çuhadaroğlu Ç, Utkusavaş A, Öztürk L, et al (2009) Effects of nasal CPAP treatment on insulin resistance, lipid profile, and plasma leptin in sleep apnea. *Lung* 187(2): 75–81.

Cuneo RC, Salomen F, Wiles CM, et al (1992) Histology of skeletal muscle in adults with GH deficiency: comparison with normal muscle and response to GH treatment. *Hormone Research* 37: 23–28.

Cuneo RC, Salomen F, Wiles CM, et al (1991) Growth hormone treatment in growth hormone-deficient adults. 1. Effects on muscle mass and strength. *Journal of Applied Physiology* 70: 688–694.

Day JL (1995) Why should patients do what we ask them to do? *Patient Education and Counselling* 26(1-3): 113–118.

de la Monte SM & Wands JR (2005) Review of insulin and insulin-like growth factor expression signalling and malfunctioning in the central nervous system: relevance to Altzheimer's disease. *Journal of Altzheimer's Disease* 7(1): 45–61.

de Jong PE, Hillege HL, Pinto-Sietsma SJ, et al (2003) Screening for microalbuminuria in the general population: a tool to detect subjects at risk for progressive renal failure in an early phase? *Nephrology, Dialysis, Transplant* 18: 10–13.

Department of Mental Diseases (1930). Annual Report of the Trustees of the Worcester State Hospital for the Year Ending November 30, 1930. Boston, 1930.

Dershowitz AM (1991) *Reversal of Fortune: Inside the von Bulow Case.* New York: Penguin Books Limited.

Diabetes Control and Complications Trial (DCCT) Research Group (1995) The relationship of glycaemic exposure (HbA1c) to the risk of development and progression of retinopathy in the Diabetes Control and Complications Trial. *Diabetes* 44(8): 968–983.

Diabetes Control and Complications Trial (DCCT) Research Group (1993) The effect of intensive treatment of diabetes on the development and progression of long-term complications in insulin-dependent diabetes mellitus. *New England Journal of Medicine* 329: 977–1034.

Diabetes UK www.diabetes.org

Diabetes UK (2008) *Cardiovascular Disease and Diabetes.* London: Diabetes UK.

Diamond MP (1998) Effects of methyltestosterone on insulin secretion and sensitivity in women. *Journal of Clinical Endocrinology and Metabolism.* 83(12): 4420–4425.

Dishman RK (1986) Exercise compliance: a new view for public health. *Physician and Sports Medicine* 14: 127–145.

Domargard A, Sarnbad S, Kroon M, et al (1999) Increased prevalence of overweight in adolescent girls with type 1 diabetes mellitus. *Paediatrics* 88: 1223–1228.

Donovan JL & Blake DR (1992) Patient non-compliance: deviance or reasoned decision-making? *Social Science Medicine* 34(5): 507–513.

Doppman JL, Chang R, Fraker DL, et al (1995) Localisation of insulinomas to regions of the pancreas by intra-arterial stimulation with calcium. *Annals of Internal Medicine* 123(4): 269–273.

Doppman JL, Chang R, Fraker Dl, et al (1995) Localisation of insulinomas to regions of the pancreas by intra-arterial stimulation with calcium. *Annals of Internal Medicine* 123(4): 269–273.

Dorkova Z, Petrasova D, Molcanyiova A, et al (2008) Effects of continuous positive airway pressure on cardiovascular risk profile in patients with severe obstructive sleep apnea and metabolic syndrome. *Chest* 134(4): 686–692.

Duchaine D (1983) *The Underground Steroid Handbook.* Canada: Ottawa, HRL Technical.

Duckworth WC, Bennett RG, Hamel FG (1998) Insulin degradation: process and potential. *Endocrinology Review* 19(5): 608–624.

Dukarm CP, Byrd RSA, Auinger P, et al (1996) Illicit substance use, gender, and the risk of violent behaviour among adolescents. *Archives of Paediatric and Adolescent Medicine*150: 797–801.

Dzaja A, Dalal MA, Himmerich H, et al (2004) Sleep enhances nocturnal plasma ghrelin levels in healthy subjects. *American Journal of Physiology* 286(6): E963–E967.

Elkin SL, Brady S, Williams IP (1997) Bodybuilders find it easy to obtain insulin to help them in training. *British Medical Journal* 314: 1280.

Elkins L (2012) My sister died because she didn't take her diabetes seriously. *Daily Mail* January 25, 2012.

Elmasry A, Janson C, Lindberg E, et al (2000) The role of habitual snoring and obesity in the development of diabetes: a 10-year follow-up study in a male population. *Journal of Internal Medicine* 248(1): 13–20.

Endler NS (1988) The origins of electro convulsive therapy. *Convulsive Therapy* 4: 5–23.

Fink M (1984) Meduna and the origins of convulsive therapy. *American Journal of Psychiatry* 141: 1034–1041.

Evans NA (2004) Current concepts in anabolic androgenic steroids. *American Journal of Sports Medicine* 32: 534–542.

Evans PJ & Lynch RM (2003) Insulin as a drug of abuse in body building. *British Journal of Sports Medicine* 37: 356–357.

Eisenberg ER & Galloway GP (2005) Anabolic androgenic steroids. In: *Substance Abuse: A Comprehensive Textbook.* Lowinson JH (ed), Ruiz RB (ed), Pennsylvania: Millman RB (ed), et al. Lippincott, Williams & Wilkins

Fainaru-Wada M & Williams L (2006) *Game of Shadows: Barry Bonds, BALCO, and the Steroid Scandal that Rocked Professional Sport.* New York: Penguin, Gotham Books.

Ferguson KL (2010) The cinema of control: on diabetic excess and illness in film. *Journal of Medical Humanities* 31(3): 183–204.

Fine RN, Sullivan EK, Tejani A (2000) The impact of recombinant human growth hormone treatment on final adult height. *Paediatric Nephrology* 14: 679-681.

Fink M (1985) *Convulsive Therapy.* New York: Raven Press.

Ford S (2008) Could Colin Norris have been stopped? *Nursing Times* 104(10) 8–9.

Friedlander A, Butterfield GE, Movnihan S, et al (2013) One year of insulin-like growth factor-1 treatment does not affect bone density, bone composition, or psychological measures in post-menopausal women. *Journal of Clinical Endocrinology and Metabolism* 86(4) http://dx.doi.org/10.1210/jcem.86.4.7377

Frith C & Johnstone E (2003) *Schizophrenia: A Very Short History.* Oxford: Oxford University Press.

Fryberg DA, John LA, Hill SA, et al (1995) Insulin and insulin-like growth factor-1 enhance human skeletal muscle protein anabolism during hyperaminoacidemia by different mechanisms. *Journal of Clinical Investigation* 96: 1722–1729.

Fryberg DA, Gelfand RA, Barrett EJ (1991) Growth hormone acutely stimulates forearm muscle protein synthesis in normal humans. *American Journal of Physiology* 260: 499–504.

210 · INSULIN USES & ABUSES

Gale SM, Castracane VD, Matzoros CS (2004) Energy homeostasis, obesity and eating disorders: recent advances in endocrinology. *Journal of Nutrition* 134(2): 295–298.

George S, Murali V, Pullickal R (2005) Review of neuroendocrine correlates of chronic opiate misuse: dysfunction and pathophysiological mechanisms. *Addictive Disorders and Their Treatment* 4(3): 99–109.

Germak JA (1996) Growth hormone therapy in children with short stature: is bigger better or achievable? *Indian Journal o Pediatrics* 63: 591-597.

Glasgow RE, Fisher EB, Anderson BJ (1999) Behavioural science in diabetes. *Diabetes Care* 22(5): 21–29.

Goebel-Fabbri AE, Fikkan J, Franko D, et al (2008) Insulin restriction and associated morbidity and mortality in women with type 1 diabetes. *Diabetes Care* 31(3): 415–419.

Goldberg GR, Prentice AM, Davies HL, et al (1988) Overnight and basal metabolic rates in men and women. *European Journal of Clinical Nutrition* 42(2): 137–144.

Golin CE, DiMatteo MR, Gelberg L (2001) The role of participation in the doctor-patient visit. *Diabetes Care* 19: 1153–1164.

Gostin LO (1980) Ethical considerations of psychosurgery: the unhappy legacy of the pre-frontal lobotomy. *Journal of Medical Ethics* 6(3): 149–154.

Gregory S & McKie L (1991) The smear test: women's views. *Nursing Standard* 5(33): 32–36.

Grylli V, Wagner G, Haffnerl-Gattermayer A, et al (2005) Disturbed eating attitudes, coping styles, and subjective quality of life in adolescents with type 1 diabetes. *Journal of Psychosomatic Research* 59: 65–72.

Gupta AK, Clark RV, Kirchner KA (1992) Effects of insulin on renal sodium excretion. *Hypertension* 19(Supplement 1): 178–182.

Haffner D & Schaefer F (2001) Does recombinant growth hormone improve adult height in children with chronic renal failure? *Seminal Nephrology* 21: 490–497.

Haibach H, Dix JD, Shah JH (1987) Homicide by insulin administration. *Journal of Forensic Science* 32: 208–216.

Hanas R (2006) *Type 1 Diabetes in Children, Adolescents and Young People.* Third edition. London: Class Publishing.

Harlan LC, Bernstein AM, Kessler LG (1991) Cervical cancer screening: who is not screened and why? *American Journal of Public Health* 81: 885–890.

Harris S (1924) Hyperinsulinism and dyinsulinism. *Journal of the American Medical Association* 83(10): 729–733.

Harrison C & Gibson A (2009) *Practical Neonatology: For MRCPCH and Beyond. London: Churchill Livingstone.*

Harvard Health Publications (2011) Controlling blood sugar levels in diabetes: how low to go? *Harvard Men's Health Watch* 15.

Hasken J, Kresl L, Nydegger T, et al (2010) Diabulimia and the role of school health personnel. *Journal of School Health* 80(10): 465–469.

Hautman P (2010) *Sweetblood.* London: Simon Schuster Children's Publishing.

Health and Social Care Information Centre (2012). www.ic.nhs.uk/article/2239/Eating-disorder-hospital-admissions-rise-by-16-percent-in-a-year

Hiestand DM, Britz P, Goldman M, et al (2006) Prevalence of risk and symptoms of sleep apnea in the US population: Results from the National Sleep Foundation Sleep in American 2005 poll. *Chest* 130(3): 780–786.

Himsworth R. (2011) Sir Harold Himsworth. *Diabetes Medicine* 28, 2, 1438–1439.

Hobbs CJ, Jones RE, Plymate SR (1996) Nandrolone, a 19-nortesterone, enhances insulin independent glucose uptake in normal men. *Journal of Clinical Endocrinology and Metabolism* 81: 1582–1585.

Holland H. (1590) *A Treatise Against Witchcraft.* Cambridge.

Holt RIG & Sonksen PH (2008) Growth hormone, IGF-1 and insulin and their abuse in sport. *British Journal of Pharmacology* 154(3): 542–556.

Huang Z & Sjöholm A (2008) Ethanol acutely stimulates islet blood flow, amplifies insulin secretion, and induces hypoglycaemia via nitric oxide and vagally mediated mechanisms. *Endocrinology* 149(1): 232–236.

Hughes R (1986) Atracurium: an overview. *British Journal of Anaesthesia* 58: supplement 1, 2S–5S.

Ip MSM, Lam B, Ng MMT, et al (2002) Obstructive sleep apnea is independently associated with insulin resistance. *American Journal of Respiratory and Critical Care Medicine* 165(5): 670–676.

Islam S (2000) *The Islets of Langerhans.* New York: Springer.

Ivy JL (1991) Muscle glycogen synthesis before and after exercise. *Sports Medicine* 11: 6–9.

Iwase H, Kobayashi M, Nakajima M, et al (2001) The ratio of insulin to C-peptide can be used to make forensic diagnosis of exogenous insulin overdose. *Forensic Science International* 115: 123–127.

Janz NK & Becker MH (1984) The Health Belief Model: a decade later. *Health Education Quarterly* 11: 147.

Jarvis S & Rubin AL (2003) *Diabetes For Dummies.* Chichester: John Wiley and Sons Limited.

Jenkins PJ (2001) Growth hormone and exercise: physiology, use and abuse. *Growth Hormone and IGF Research* 11(supplement A): S71–S77.

Jennum P, Schultz-Larsen K, Christensen N (1993) Snoring, sympathetic activity and cardiovascular risk factors in a 70 year old population. *European Journal of Epidemiology* 9(5): 477–482.

Johna S & Schein M (2003) *The Memoirs of Allen Oldfather Whipple: The Man Behind the Whipple Operation.* Wiltshire: TFM Publishing Limited.

JBDS (2010) Joint British Diabetes Society guidelines for the management of diabetic ketoacidosis in adults. Available at www.diabets.nhs.uk

JDRF (Juvenile Diabetes Research Foundation www.jdrf.org

Jones CA, Francis ME, Eberhardt MS, et al (2002) Microalbuminuria in the US population: Third National Health and Nutrition Survey. *American Journal of Kidney Disease* 39: 445–459.

Katz J & Peberdy A (1997) *Promoting Health, Knowledge and Practice.* Basingstoke and London: McMillan Press Limited.

Katsilambros N, Kanka-Gantenbein C, Liatis S, et al (2011) *Diabetic Emergencies and Clinical Management.* Chichester, West Sussex: Wiley-Blackwell.

Kaufman DM (2007) *Clinical Neurology for Psychiatrists.* Sixth edition, Philadelphia: Saunders.

Kelly SD, Howe CJ, Hendler JP, et al (2005) Disordered eating behaviours in youth with type 1 diabetes. *The Diabetes Educator* 31(4): 572–587.

Khaleeli AA, Levy RD, Edwards RH, et al (1984) The neuromuscular features of acromegaly: a clinical and pathological study. *Journal of Neurological and Neurosurgical Psychiatry* 47: 1009–1015.

Krentz AJ & Hitman GA (2011) Sir Harold Himsworth and insulin insensitivity 75 years on. *Diabetes Medicine* 28, 2, 1435.

Krishmamoorthy S, Narain R, Creamer J (2009) Unusual presentation of thyrotoxicosis as complete heart block and renal failure: a case report. *Journal of Medical Case Reports* 3: 9303.

Kutscher EC, Lund BC, Perry PJ (2002) Anabolic steroids: a review for the physician. *Sports Medicine* 32: 285–296.

Larranaga A, Docet MF, Garcia-Mayor RV (2011) Disordered eating in type 1 diabetes patients. *World Journal of Diabetes* 2: 189–195.

Leger J, Garel C, Fjellstad-Paulsen A, et al (1998) Human growth factor treatment of short- stature children small for gestational age: effect on muscle and adipose tissue mass during a 3-year treatment period and after 1 year's withdrawal. *Journal of Clinical Endocrinology and Metabolism* 83: 3512–3516.

Lewis DA & Levitt P (2002) Schizophrenia as a disorder of natural development. *Annual Review of Neuroscience* 25: 409–432.

Lifshutz JE (1954) Insulin coma therapy. *American Journal of Psychiatry* 110:466–469.

Lindberg E, Berne C, Franklin KA, et al (2007) Snoring and daytime sleepiness as risk factors for hypertension and diabetes in women – a population-based study. *Respiratory Medicine* 101(6): 1283–1290.

Liow RT & Tavares S (1995) Bilateral rupture of the quadriceps tendon associated with anabolic steroids. *British Journal of Sports Medicine* 29: 77–79.

Loveday J (1991) *Davies' Medical Terminology, A Guide to Current Usage.* Oxford: Butterworth-Heinemann.

Lukas SE (2003) The pharmacology of steroids. In: *Principles of Addiction Medicine* Graham AW (ed), Schultz TK (ed), and Mayo-Smith MF (ed), et al. American Society of Addiction Medicine, 305–321.

Lustman PJ, Anderson RJ, Freedland KE, et al (2000) Depression and poor glycaemic control: a meta-analytic review of the literature. *Diabetes Care* 23: 934–942.

Lyssenko V, Nagorny CLF, Erdos MR, et al (2009) Common variant in MTNR1B associated with increased risk of type 2 diabetes and impaired early insulin secretion. *Nature Genetics* 41(1): 82–88.

MacIsaac RJ & Watts GF (2005) Diabetes and the Kidneys. In: Shaw KM and Cummings MH (eds) *Diabetes Chronic Complications,* second edition, Chichester: John Wiley and Sons.

Mackay RP (1965) Ladislas Joseph Meduna 1896–1965. *Recent Advances in Biological Psychiatry* 8: 357–358.

Madea B & Rödig A (2006) Time of death dependent criteria in vitreous humour: accuracy of estimating the time since death. *Forensic Science International* 164 (2-3): 87–92.

Mallon L, Broman J-E, Hetta J (2005) High incidence of diabetes in men with sleep complaints or sleep duration: a 12-year follow-up study of a middle-aged population. *Diabetes Care* 28(11): 2762–2767.

Mankell H (2012) *One Step Behind.* New York: Vintage Books.

Markowitz JT, Antisdel JE, Butler DA, et al (2010) Brief screening tool for disordered eating in diabetes. *Diabetes Care* 33(3): 495–500.

Marks V & Richmond C (2008a) Kenneth Barlow: the first documented case of murder by insulin. *Journal of the Royal Society of Medicine* 101(1): 19–21.

Marks V & Richmond C (2008b) William Archerd: a serial matrimonial killer. *Journal of the Royal Society of Medicine* 101(2): 63–66.

Marks V & Richmond C (2008c) Colin Bouwer: Professor of Psychology and Murderer. *Royal Society of Medicine* 101(8): 400–408.

Marks V & Richmond C (2007) *Insulin Murders, True Life Cases.* London: The Royal Society of Medicine Press Limited.

Marks V (2006) Hypoglycaemia: insulin and conflicts with the law. *British Journal of Diabetes and Vascular Disease* 6: 281–185.

Marks V (2005) Hypo: accidents and murder, part 2. *Practical Diabetes* 22(9): 355–358.

Marks V & Teale JD (2001) Hypoglycaemic disorders. *Clinical Laboratory Medicine* 21: 79–97.

Marks V (1993) Forensic aspects of hypoglycaemia. In Frier B & Fisher M (eds.) *Hypoglycaemia and Diabetes.* London: Edward Arnold.

Marks V (1992) Recognition and differential diagnosis of spontaneous hypoglycaemia. *Clinical Endocrinology* 37(4): 309–316.

Marks V & Medd WE (1964) Alcohol-induced hypoglycaemia. *British Journal of Psychiatry* 110: 228–232.

Marteau TM & Kinmouth AL (1988) Doctors' beliefs about diabetes: a comparison of hospital and community doctors. *British Journal of Clinical Psychology* 27: 181–183.

Marwood SF (1973) Diabetes mellitus – some reflections. *Journal of the Royal College of General Practitioners* 23, 38.

Mazze R, Lucido D, Shamoon H (1984) Psychological and social correlates of glycaemic control. *Diabetes Care* 7: 360-366.

McCaul KD, Schroeder DM, Reid PA (1996) Brest cancer worry and screening: some prospective data. *Health Psychology* 15:430–433.

McCrimmon RJ & Frier BM (1994) Hypoglycaemia, the most feared complication of insulin therapy. *Diabetes Metabolism* 20: 503–512.

Miller FP, Vandrome A, McBrewster J (2009) *Lysosomal Storage Disease.* Alphascript Publishing, Beau Bassin: Mauritius.

Mohamed Q, Gillies MC, Wong TY (2007) Management of diabetic retinopathy. *Journal of the American Medical Association* 298, 8, 902–916.

Moore R (2013) *The Dirtiest Race in History: Ben Johnson, Carl Lewis, and the 1988 Olympic 100 metres Final.* London: Bloomsbury, Wisden.

Morris C & McAllister C (2005) Etomidate for emergency anaesthesia: mad, bad and dangerous to know? *Anaesthesia* 60(8): 737–740.

Mukhapadyay R (2007) Catching doping athletes. *Analytical Chemistry* 5522–5528.

Nasar S (1998) *A Beautiful Mind.* New York: Simon and Schster.

National Diabetes Inpatient Audit (2011) https://catalogue.ic.nhs.uk/publications/clinical/diabetes/nati-diab-inp-audi-11/nati-diab-inp-audi-11-nat-rep-pdf

National Eating Disorders Association

www.nationaleatingdisorders.org

National Institute for Health and Care Excellence (2004) CG9: Eating disorders: core interventions in the treatment and management of anorexia nervosa, bulimia nervosa and related eating disorders. http://publications.nice.org.uk/eating-disorders-cg9

National Paediatric Diabetes Audit (2011) www.hqip.org.uk/assests/NCAPOP-Library/NCAPOP-2012-13/Dabetes-Paediatric-Audit-Report-pub-2012.pdf

Neumark-Sztainer D (2002) Weight control practices and disordered eating behaviours among adolescent females and males with type 1 diabetes. *Diabetes Care* 25: 1289–1296.

Nash JF (2007) *The Essential John Nash.* New Jersey: Princeton University Press.

Norton PG & Dunn EV (1985) Snoring as a risk factor for disease: an epidemiological survey. *British Journal of Medicine* 291(6496): 30–32.

Olmstead MP, Colton PA, Daneman D, et al (2008) Predictions of the onset of disturbed eating behaviour in adolescent girls with type 1 diabetes. *Diabetes Care* 31(10): 1978–1982.

Okada M, Takamizawa A, Tsushima K, et al (2006) Relationship between sleep-disordered breathing and lifestyle-related illness in subjects who have undergone health screening. *Internal Medicine* 45(15): 891–896.

Patti ME, McMahon G, Mun EC (2005) Severe hypoglycaemic post-gastric bypass requiring partial pancreatectomy: evidence for inappropriate insulin secretion and islet hyperplasia. *Diabetologia* 48(11): 2236–2240.

Patrick AW & Campbell IW (1990) Fatal hypoglycaemia in insulin-treated diabetes mellitus: clinical features and neuropathological changes. *Diabetes Medicine* 7: 349–354.

Pearce JMS (2008) Leopold Auenbrugger: camphor-induced epilepsy – remedy for manic psychosis. *European Neurology* 59 (1-2): 105–107.

Perheetupa J, Raivio KO, Nikkilä EA (2009) Hereditary fructose intolerance. *Acta Medica Scandinavia* 192, S542, 65–75.

Peveler RC, Bryden KS, Neil AW, et al (2005) The relationship of disordered eating habits and attitudes to clinical outcomes in young adult females with type 1 diabetes. *Diabetes Care* 28(1): 84–88.

Pitchess PJ (1969) Proof of murder by insulin – a medico-legal first. *FBI Law Bulletin* January 16–19.

Pope HG & Katz DL (1994) Psychiatric and medical effects of anabolic androgenic steroid use: a controlled study of 160 athletes. *Archives of General Psychiatry* 51: 375–382.

Pope HG & Katz DL (1988) Affective and psychotic symptoms associated with anabolic steroid use. *American Journal of Psychiatry* 147: 487–490.

Prochaska JP & DiClemente CC (1984) *The Trantheoretical Approach: Crossing Traditional Boundaries of Change.* Homewood, Illinois: Don Jones/Irwin.

Puccio T (1995) *In the Name of the Law: Confessions of a Trial Lawyer.* New York: Random House.

Punjabi NM, Sorkin JD, Katzel LI, et al (2002) Sleep-disordered breathing and insulin resistance in middle-aged and overweight men. *American Journal of Respiratory and Critical Care Medicine* 165(5): 77–82.

Punjabi NM, Shahar E, Redline S, et al (2004) Sleep-disordered breathing, glucose intolerance, and insulin resistance. *American Journal of Epidemiology* 160(6): 521–530.

Randle PJ, Garland PB, Newholme EA, et al (1965) The glucose fatty acids cycle in obesity and maturity-onset diabetes mellitus. *Annals of the New York Academy of Sciences* 131: 324–333.

Rashid H, Ormerod S, Day E (2007) Anabolic androgenic steroids: what the psychiatrist needs to know. *Advances in Psychiatric Treatment* 13: 203–211.

Renko A-K, Hiltunen L, Laakso M, et al (2005) The relationship of glucose tolerance to sleep disorders and daytime sleepiness. *Diabetes Research and Clinical Practice* 67(1): 84–91.

Rennie MJ (2003) Claims for the anabolic effects of growth hormone: a case of the Emperor's new clothes? *British Journal of Sports Medicine* 37: 100–105.

Rich JD, Dickinson BP, Merriman NA, et al (1998) Insulin use by bodybuilders. *Journal of the American Medical Association* 279: 1613.

Rives JD, Shepard RM (1951) Thyroid crisis. *American Surgery* 17: 406–418.

Robertson RP, Holman TV, Genuth S (1998) Pancreas transplantation for type 1 diabetes – a summation. *The Journal of Clinical Endocrinology & Metabolism* 83(6): 1868–1874.

Rosin S (1991) Pilocarpine. A miotic of choice in the treatment of glaucoma has passed 110 years of use. *Oflalmologia* 35(1): 53–55.

Ross JR & Malzberg (1939) A review of the results of pharmacological shock therapy and the metrazol convulsive therapy in New York. *American Psychiatric Association* 96: 297–316.

Rossing P, Andersen H, Hesselholdt L, et al (2001) Attitudes towards diabetes and its care: evaluation before, immediately post-course and > 1 year after a practical interventional inter-disciplinary course for diabetes teams. *Practical Diabetes International* 18(2): 345–349.

Russell RC (2012) *Diabetic Ketoacidosis.* Seattle, Washington: VSD Publications.

Ruth-Sahd LA, Schneider M, Haagen B (2010) What is diabulimia? *Nursing in Critical Care* 5(4): 40–44.

Ruth-Sahd LA, Schneider M, Haagen B (2009) Diabulimia: what is it and how to recognise it in critical care. *Dimensions of Critical Care Nursing* 28(4): 147–153.

Rydall AC, Rodin GM, Olmstead MP, et al (1997) Disordered eating behaviour and microvascular complications in young women with insulin dependent diabetes mellitus. *New England Journal of Medicine* 336: 1849–1854.

Sakel M (1930) Insulin in the treatment of symptoms accompanying withdrawal of morphine. *Deutsche Meziniche Wochenschnft* LVI 1777.

Sakel M (1937a) Origins and nature of hypoglycaemic therapy of psychosis. *Achieves of Neurology and Psychiatry* 38: 188–203.

Sakel M (1937b) The methodical use of hypoglycaemia in the treatment of psychoses. *American Journal of Psychiatry* 151(supplement 6): 240–247.

Sakel M (1956) Sakel shock treatment. In *The Great Physiological Therapies in Psychiatry: A Historical Perspective.* AM Sackler (Ed) New York: Harper & Brothers.

Salomon F, Cuneo R, Hesp R, et al (1989) The effects of treatment with recombinant human growth hormone on body composition and metabolism in adults with growth hormone deficiency. *New England Journal of Medicine* 321: 1797–1803.

Savage MW, Dhatariya KK, Kilvert A et al (2011) Joint British Diabetes Societies guidelines for the management of diabetic ketoacidosis. *Diabetic Medicine* 28: 508–515.

Schafer EA (1916) *The Endocrine Organs – An Introduction to the Study of Internal Secretions.* London: Longman, Green and Co.

Schoeller DA, Cella LK, Sinha MK, et al (1997) Entrainment of the diurnal level of plasma leptin to meal timing. *Journal of Clinical Investigation* 100(7): 1882–1887.

Service GL, Thompson GB, Service FJ, et al (2005) Hyperinsulineamic hypooglycaemia with Nesidioblastosis after gastric-bypass surgery. *New England Journal of Medicine* 353(3): 249–254.

Shaban C (2013) Diabulimia: mental health condition or media hyperbole? *Practical Diabetes* 30(3): 104–105a.

Sharma S & Kavuru M (2010) Sleep and metabolism: overview. *International Journal of Endocrinology.* Published online doi: 10.1155/2010/270832

Shaw A & Favazza A (2010) Insulin under-dosing and omission should be included in DSM-V criteria for bulimia nervosa (letter to the editor). *Journal of Neuropsychiatry and Clinical Neuroscience* 22(3): 352.

Shaw KM (ed) & Cummings MH (ed) (2005) *Diabetes: Chronic Complications.* Second edition, Chichester: John Wiley and Sons Limited.

Shigeta H, Shigeta M, Nakazawa A, et al (2001) Lifestyle , obesity and insulin resistance. *Diabetes Care* 24(3): 608.

Shotliff K & Duncan G (2005) Diabetes and the Eye. In: Shaw KM & Cummings MH (eds) *Diabetes Complications*, second edition, Chichester: John Wiley and Sons.

Sidaway AN & Curry KM (1991) Non-invasive evaluation of the lower extremity arterial system. In: Frykberg RG (ed) *The High Risk Foot in Diabetes Mellitus.* Edinburgh: Churchill Livingstone.

Siegel JM (2003) Why we sleep. *Scientific American* 289(5): 92–97.

Singa A, Formica C, Tsalamandris C, et al (1996) Effect of insulin on body composition in patients with insulin-dependent and non-insulin dependent diabetes. *Diabetic Medicine* 13: 40–46.

Skårberg K, Nyberg F, Engström I (2008) The development of multi-drug use among anabolic-androgenic steroid users: six subjective case reports. *Substance Abuse Treatment, Prevention, and Policy* 3: 24–34.

Slater E & Sargeant W (1944) The insulin treatment of schizophrenia. In: *An Introduction to Physical Methods of Treatment in Psychiatry.* First edition, Edinburgh E & S, Livingstone.

Smith FM, Latchford GJ, Hall RM, et al (2008) Do chronic medical conditions increase the risk of eating disorder? A cross-sectional investigation of eating pathology in adolescent females with scoliosis and diabetes. *Journal of Adolescent Health* 42: 58–63.

Sonksen PH (2001) Insulin, growth hormone and sport. *Journal of Endocrinology* 170: 13–25.

Sonksen PH & Sonksen J (2000) Insulin: Understanding its action in health and disease. *Journal of Anaesthesia* 85(1): 69–79.

Spiegel K, Leprolt R, Van Cauter E (2005) Metabolic and endocrine changes. In Kushida C (ed) *Sleep Deprivation: Basic Science, Physiology and Behaviour.* Volume 192, New York, USA, Marcel Dekker, pp 293–318.

Spiegel K, Leproult R, L'Hermite-Balériax M, et al (2004a) Leptin levels are dependent on sleep duration: relationships with sympathovagal balance, carbohydrate regulation, cortisol, and thyrotropin. *Journal of Clinical Endocrinology and Metabolism* 89(11): 5762–5771.

Spiegel K, Tasali E, Penev P, et al (2004b) Brief communication: sleep curtailment in healthy young men is associated with decreased leptin levels, elevated ghrelin levels and feelings of hunger in normal-weight healthy men. *Annals of Internal Medicine* 141(11): 846–850.

Spiegel K, Leprolt R, Colecchia FF, et al (2000) Adaptation of the 24-h growth hormone profile to a state of sleep debt. *American Journal of Physiology* 279(3): R864–R833.

Stabler B, Lane JD, Ross SL, et al (1988) Behaviour patters and chronic glycaemic control in individuals with IDDM. *Diabetes Care* 11: 361–362.

Starkey K & Wade T (2010) Disordered eating in girls with type 1 diabetes: examining directions for prevention. *Clinical Psychologists* 14(1): 2–9.

Steen E, Terry BM, Rivera EJ, et al (2005) Impaired insulin and insulin-like growth factor expression and signalling in Alzheimer's disease. *Journal of Altzheimer's Disease* 7(1): 63–80.

Stephens JH, Richard P, McHugh PR (2000) Long-term follow-up of patients with a diagnosis of paranoid state and hospitalized, 1913 to 1940. *Journal Nervous Mental Diseases* 188: 202–208.

Su T, Pagliaro M, Schmidt P, et al (1993) Neuropsychiatric effects of anabolic steroids in male normal volunteers. *Journal of the American Medical Association* 269: 2760–2764.

Sweetman SC (2009) (ed.) *Martindale: The Complete Drug Reference.* 36th edition, London: Pharmaceutical Press.

Taheri S, Lin L, Austin D, et al (2004) Short sleep duration is associated with reduced leptin, elevated ghrelin, and increased boxy mass index. *PloS Medicine* 1(3): e62.

Talbot F & Nouwen A (2000) A review of the relationship between depression and diabetes in adults: is there a link? *Diabetes Care* 23: 1556–1562.

Tappin JW, Pollard J, Bechett EA (1980) Method of measuring shear forces on the sole of the foot. *Clinical Physical & Physiological Measurement* 1: 83–85.

Tasker AP, Gibson L, Franklin V, et al (2007) What is the frequency of mild symptomatic hypoglycaemia in the young: assessment by novel mobile phone technology and computer based interviewing. *Paediatric Diabetes* 8(1): 15–20.

The American Psychiatric Association

www.psch.org

The American Psychological Association

www.apa.org

The Behavioural Diabetes Institute

www.behaviouraldiabetesinstitute.org

Thevis M, Thomas A, Delahaut P, et al (2006) Doping control analysis of intact rapid-acting insulin analogues in human urine by liquid chromatography-tandem mass spectrometry. *Analytical Chemistry* 78(6): 1897–1903.

Thomas A, Thevis M, Delehaut P, et al (2007) Mass spectromic identification of degradation products of insulin and its long-acting analogues in human urine for doping control purposes. *Analytical Chemistry* 79(6): 2518–2524.

Tierney S, Deaton C, Whitehead J (2008) Caring for people with type 1 diabetes mellitus engaging in disturbed eating or weight control: a qualitative study of practitioners' attitudes and practices. *Journal of Clinical Nursing* 18: 384–390.

Tortora GJ & Grabowski SR (1993) *Principles of Anatomy and Physiology.* Seventh edition, New York: Harper Collins College Publishers.

Trennel MI (2007) Sleep and metabolic control: waking into a problem? *Clinical and Experimental Pharmacology* 34(1-2): 2–3.

Tricker R, O'Neill MR, Cook D (1989) The incidence of anabolic steroid use among competitive body builders. *Journal of Drug Education* 19: 313–325.

UK Prospective Diabetes Study Group (1998) Tight blood pressure control and risk of macro-vascular and microvascular complications in type 2 diabetes (UKPDS 38). *British Medical Journal* 317: 703–712.

Urhausen A, Albers T, Kindermann W (2004) Are the cardiac effects of anabolic steroids reversible? *Heart* 90: 496–501.

Valcavi R, Menozzi C, Roti E, et al (1992) Sinus node function in hyperthyroid patients. *Journal of Clinical Endocrinology and Metabolism* 75(1): 239–242.

Van Cauter E, Polonsky KS, Scheen AJ (1997) Roles of circadian rhythmicity and sleep in human glucose regulation. *Endocrine Reviews* 18(5): 716–738.

Van Cauter E, Kerkhofs M, Caufriez A, et al (1992) A quantitative estimation of growth hormone secretion in normal man: reproducibility and relation to time by day. *Journal of Clinical Endocrinology and Metabolism* 74(6): 1441–1450.

Vanholder R, Massy Z, Argiles A, et al. (2005) Chronic kidney disease as cause of cardiovascular morbidity and mortality. *Nephrology, Dialysis and Transplant* 20, 6. 1048–1056.

Valenstein ES (1986) *Great and Desperate Cures: The Rise and Decline of Psychosurgery* **psychosurgery** *Treatment of psychosis or other mental disorders by means of brain surgery. The first such technique was the prefrontal lobotomy. Fairly common from the 1930s through the 1950s, lobotomy reduced neurotic symptoms such as agitation and aggressiveness but also and Other Radical Treatments for Mental Illness.* New York: Basic Books.

Vgontzas AN, Papanicolaou DA, Bixler EO, et al (2000) Sleep apnea and daytime sleepiness and fatigue: relation to visceral obesity, insulin resistance, and hypercytokinemia. *Journal of Clinical Endocrinology and Metabolism* 85(3): 1151–1158.

Vriesendorp T, van Santen S, DeVries J, et al (2006) Predisposing factors for hypoglycaemia in the intensive care unit. *Critical Care Medicine* 34(1): 96–101.

Wark P (2007) Diabulimia: the new threat. *The Times* July 15, 2007.

Warren RE, Zammitt NN, Deary IJ, et al (2007) The effects of active hypoglycaemia on memory acquisition and recall and prospective memory in type 1 diabetes. *Diabetologia* 50(1): 178–185.

Wax R (2013) *Sane New World: Taming The Mind.* Croydon, UK: Hodder & Stoughton.

Weitz D (2004) *Insulin Shock – A Survivor's Guide to Psychiatric Torture.* psychrights.org/stories/insulin-shock-A-Survivors-Account.pdf

West SD, Nicoll DJ, Wallace TM, et al (2007) Effect of CPAP on insulin resistance and HbA1c in men with obstructive sleep apnea and Type 2 diabetes. *Thorax* 62(11): 969–974.

Whitaker R (2010) *Mad in America: Bad Science, Bad Medicine, and Enduring Mistreatment of the Mentally Ill.* New York: Perseus, Basic Books.

Wilson VL (2013) Type 2 diabetes in children and adolescents: a growing epidemic. *Nursing Children and Young People* 25(2): 14–17.

Wilson VL (2012) Reflections on reducing insulin to lose weight. *Nursing Times* 108(43): 21–15.

Wilson VL (2011) Non-diabetic hypoglycaemia: causes and pathophysiology. *Nursing Standard* 25(46): 35–40

Wilson VL (2010) Students managing type 1 diabetes. *Paediatric Nursing* 22(10): 25–18

Wilson VL (2009) Behavioural change in type 1 diabetes: why and how? *Health Education Journal* 68(4): 320–327.

Wilson VL (2003) Insulin pump therapy: a patient's perspective. *Diabetes and Primary Care* 5(3): 132–136

Wootton D (2006) *Bad Medicine: Doctors Doing Harm Since Hippocrates.* New York: Oxford University Press.

World Health Organisation, (2011) *Diabetes,* factsheet number 312. Geneva: World Health Organisation.

Wraight W (1983) *The von Bulow Affair.* New York: Delacote Press.

Wright J, Ruck K, Rabbitts R et al (2009) Diabetic ketoacidosis (DKA) in Birmingham, UK, 2000–2009: an evaluation of risk factors for recurrence and mortality. *British Journal of Diabetes and Vascular Disease* 9: 278–282.

Yorker BC, Kizer KW, Lampe P, et al (2006) Serial murder by healthcare professionals. *Journal of Forensic Sciences*51(6): 1362–1371.

Young T, Peppard PE, Gottlieb DJ (2002) Epidemiology of obstructive sleep apnea: a population health perspective. *American Journal of Respiratory and Critical Care Medicine* 165(9): 1217–1239.

Young V, Eiser C, Johnson B, et al (2013) Eating problems in adolescents with type 1 diabetes: a systematic review with meta-analysis. *Diabetes Medicine* 30: 189–198.

Zou L, Yuan H, Pei X, et al (2008) Diffusion tensor imaging study of the anterior limb of internal capsules in neuroleptic-naive schizophrenia. *Academic Radiology* 285–289.

# INDEX

www.ingramcontent.com/pod-product-compliance
Lightning Source LLC
Chambersburg PA
CBHW061726270326
41928CB00011B/2129